D1267570

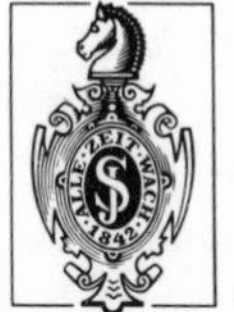
ALLE ZEIT WACH
1842

The publication of this book was made possible
through the financial support of
Bayer AG, Leverkusen.

FRANÇOIS DU PORT

THE DECADE OF MEDICINE

OR

The Physician of the Rich and the Poor

in which all the Signs, Causes and Remedies of Disease Are Clearly Expounded

Edited by H. Diehl

Original Edition Printed in 1694

Springer-Verlag
Berlin Heidelberg New York
Paris London Tokyo

HELMUT DIEHL, Droste-Hülshoff-Straße 6,
D-5000 Köln 40, FRG

Title of the Original edition: La Décade de Médecine ou Le Médecin des Riches et de Pauvres. Composé en Vers Latins par FRANÇOIS DU PORT, Médecin de Paris. Nouvellement mis en Vers François par Mr. DU FOUR, Docteur en Médecine, Conseiller & Médecin ordinaire du Roy.
1694 LAURENT D'HOURY, Paris

ISBN 3-540-19291-3 Springer-Verlag Berlin Heidelberg New York
ISBN 0-387-19291-3 Springer-Verlag New York Berlin Heidelberg

Printed in Germany

Typesetting, printing and bookbinding:
Universitätsdruckerei H. Stürtz AG, Würzburg

2125/3114-543210

Preface

The purpose of this book is to give the reader an impression of medical science in seventeenth-century France. The French physician FRANÇOIS DU PORT was the actual author of the book ›La Décade de Médecine ou Le Médecin des Riches et des Pauvres‹. Working for thirty years as a country doctor enabled him to report the symptoms and causes of different diseases, and during the reign of LOUIS XIII (1601–1643), he recorded his experiences in Latin verse. In 1691, the adviser and official physician to LOUIS XIV DU FOUR acquired the rights to DU PORT's book: he transcribed the doctor's experiences into French verse and in 1694, in Paris, ›La Décade de Médecine ou Le Médecin des Riches et des Pauvres‹ was published in Latin and French verse.

In 1980, whilst staying in Avignon, France, M. DIEHL chanced upon a copy of this edition, which was then exactly 286 years old. Her father, H. DIEHL, was fascinated by the possibility of gaining an insight into the diagnostic and therapeutic practices of the 17th century in this unusual way. As soon as he returned home, he started translating the book into German: It is divided into 10 sections with 253 chapters and approximately 500 pages. The book was translated into English by Dr. DAVID LE VAY, Wadhurst, England, in 1988.

GEORG HARTMANN

BOOK ONE

Preface

I shall examine the different springs and the most hidden ills that our bodies contain. I intend to list their causes and their signs, to vanquish them by signal remedies. O God! that's my intent, second my plan; accord Thy poet superhuman aid. For our small body is the microcosm: it understands what is seen in air, on earth, at sea, yet without the Creator, all that is seen there is not to be conceived even by the greatest spirits. You only give the healing virtue to our plants; and for our pressing ills You draw on the seas, the earth and heavens for that which gives men health; and You extend to us these presents from Your hand. Now I commence, inspire my courage and let me fortunately complete this work.

CHAPTER I

The Signs and Causes of Perfect Health

Who would descend to Apollo's secret cave, to take a draught from the fountain-head and deal with the symptoms of the human body's ills, must first enquire about the signs and causes of health itself. Therefore a florid complexion, ease of breathing and coordinated motion, a pulse that is never felt to be irregular and welcome peaceful slumber: the bladder's fluid habitually of middling consistence and its colour a diffused yellow, likewise what is naturally extruded from the bowel is soft and formed and inoffensive: in sum, when every function is active in the body without pain, these are signs of health, the opposite are those of disease. And the liver is the source of this, by making the good blood which nourishes all parts.

CHAPTER II

The Signs and Causes of Euaemia, or Good Blood, and of Polyaemia or Plethora

When the blood is in good state and the humours symmetrical, then the complexion is pleasing, changing from red to snowy white, mixing the redness of the rose with the candour of the lily, the mind is tranquil and the body full of vigour, the images of dreams peaceful and joyous. The veins are full, and full the arteries that pulsing throb, the flesh ruddy and solid un-

less it become corrupted. But when there is plethora, suffering brings dull torpor, the blood tightly distends the veins, sickness lies heavy on the limbs. The sweat flows apace, sleep is heavy and profound, the complexion rubicund, swollen and purple, the pulse habitually full and strong and the least effort causes breathlessness. The arms, the legs, the hands, the very flesh, are swollen. Bleeding relieves, and restraint in food and drink. Prone to this humour is the young man, merry and rubicund, of easy habit, naturally inclined to food, whose vessels swell with profound sleep, not given to exercise, with healthy heart and liver as the source and flow of blood: springtime and the west wind add to this distress, and even wine.

CHAPTER III

The Signs and Causes of Excessive Yellow Bile

When there is excess of bile the jaundice is of the same colour, the skin dry and irritable and burning when touched with the hand, the flesh beneath is wasted and the mood savage and vengeful with sudden fits of rage, and sleep is short and unquiet, and the artery at the wrist is full, frequent and bounding. The urine flows bitter and yellow from the kidneys, with only minimal sediment. If pustules mar the skin and there is vomiting, or the bowel's motions are stinking faeces, it all has the same yellow lustre. Cold and damp are helpful, and the voiding of the bile comforting and useful. Prone to the bile

is he who, always wakeful, eats but little while supping on sorrows: a man, hot and dry by temperament and given to fits of rage, when young, who labours to excess yet cannot usually, by nature or by art, evade the torment of the bile.

CHAPTER IV

The Signs and Causes of Overpowering Melancholy

Sombre is the hue of the man suffused with blackish bile, his body thin and dry and of meagre bulk. His aspect is frightful, his mind wanders and he says little, his spirit gloomy with sorrows, anxiety and horror that come at dead of night with ideas that disturb his mournful mind. Often he is as hungry as a dog, yet with appetite unsated he belches acid, his pulse is slow and infrequent, while the fluid leaving the kidneys is thin and pale, occasionally thick and foul and blackish. The skin is black with vitiligo or speckled with scurf, piles emerge at the anus or varices in the leg, and there may be cancer in the breast. Food causing flatulence is noxious. The juice of meat is excellent, and clear wine diluted thin; and drugs are helpful if but they purge the black humour. Whoever is dry and cold, with liver, heart and spleen weak and obstructed, has dark abundant humour: severe care and vigilance oppress the studious, the mind is seized and gapes at things in terror. And this applies to those who drink coarse red wine, who cram themselves with

meat preserved in salt, who are without piles or varicosities, whose womb is without menses but has foul discharge, especially those desperate from this: or if the year is cold, or hot and dry, or the autumn capricious.

CHAPTER V

The Signs and Causes of Excess of Phlegm

He who is oppressed with phlegm is pale of face and body, sometimes livid or of leaden colour, is foully crammed, his skin is soft and cold to the touch, his body fleshy and swollen with loose fat, the pulse small and soft and beating slow: what flows from the bladder is livid or else pale, now thin, now dirty or turbid with coarse deposit. He vomits phlegm and passes it below, but those subject to the phlegm do better if it is exuded from the moist body. The mind is sluggish, the senses heavy and sleep profound. His dreams are of water and balmy hyperborean climate, he is tardy in the performance of his duties. Useful it is for sufferers if the phlegm is expelled by the natural pathways, and hot food and drink are helpful. It is a fact that liver, heart and brain, and cold, are known as frequent causes of the phlegm, as are an idle life and frequent slumber and drinking too much water, and the weakness of age, gluttony and vexation. And if, in this disease, the phlegm is no longer expelled by nose and bowel, sputum and vomit, then it affects the body as a whole.

CHAPTER VI

The Signs and Causes of the Aqueous Humour

When watery fluid is dominant, the complexion is florid or else there is ghastly pallor, and the hands and feet are swollen so as to pit with pressure of the finger just as happens with the disease called the hydrops. The abdomen swells intermittently and splashes with the fluid moving to and fro. The aqueous humour is excreted by the kidneys and passed raw by the bowel. The pulse is soft and slow, also small and rare and weak, and fluid moistens the pale skin. There is much sputum but without cough, the mind heavy and drowsy, and the excess phlegm makes for apathy. The cause of this ill is a hard or obstructed liver, or a spleen that is also feeble and obstructed or as scirrhous as the liver, or a perverse stomach unable to manage food that is cold or moist with excessive drinking, something that is likely to happen in old age. Should the customary sweat or watery flux from the bowel be arrested, or discharge of urine not be the response to drinking, the fluid wells up and there is hydrops.

CHAPTER VII

The Signs and Causes of Severe Flatulence

Overpowering flatulence, wandering throughout the body, presses painfully on the stomach, and excites frequent cracking and ringing

in the ears. A limb may writhe in spasm, and sleep brings ideas of rapid motion through the air, like lightning, all violent confusion. And the heat produced by a crude humour causes this flatulence, unrefreshing and enfeebling, for the body is distended in its cavities as the earth's hollows confine the winds.

CHAPTER VIII

The Signs and Causes of Impending Disease

If the body is habitually lean, or fat, too hot or heavy, or sleep is so disturbed that brief slumber makes one drowsy: or the skin is foully ulcerated, the chest and neck and knees all wet with sweat, languour of spirit weakening the body; and if there is pain in the eyes and breast and heart or vessels of the head, the limbs possessed by shivering, or if one is heavy-hearted and yawns ever and again; then it is sure that sickness is already here or will be soon: the cause of which is excess of noxious humour.

CHAPTER IX

The Signs and Causes of an Attack of Fever

When fever is on its way the body is chill and overcome by cold, the nose is stiffened and there is repeated cough, and the strength fails. There is headache, vomiting and besetting drowsiness, the pulse is obscure, its beat less marked, and from time to time one yawns with arms out-

stretched. The cause is that heat that suddenly returns, redoubling the heat within and baring the outer parts to cold.

CHAPTER X

The Signs and Causes of Increasing Fever

The increase comes when absent fever gives way to tepid warmth, and the pulse, formerly so equable, now proves irregular and forceful. This is what explains the heat within that gradually extends without, by this the pulse is made to beat and warmth expelled along the limbs.

CHAPTER XI

The Signs and Causes of the Febrile State

But should the heat extend apace throughout the body, the symptoms are more marked than they were before: then death ensues, or recovery if the strength exists, for both forms of heat have their effect. Externally, if there is little noxious humour to affect the body, it vanishes: but if it is abundant, both heat and nature lose their vigour.

CHAPTER XII

The General Signs and Causes of Fever

Here there is headache and the tongue is dry and rough: there is thirst and heat and hiccough, nausea and anxiety, vomiting, weakness

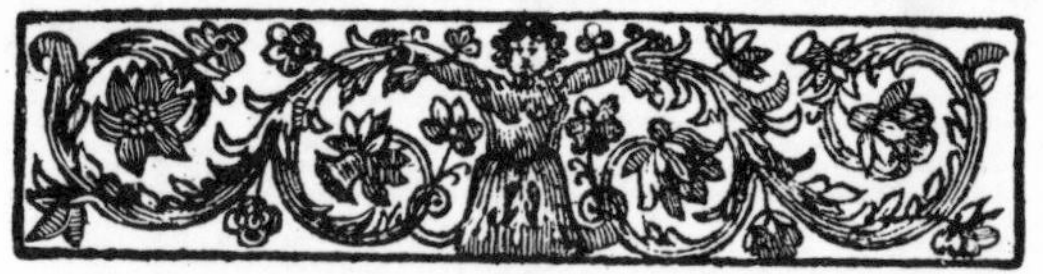

THE DECADE OF MEDICINE

OR

The Physician of the Rich and the Poor

in which all the Signs, Causes and Remedies of Diseases Are Clearly Expounded

Composed in Latin verse by

FRANÇOIS DU PORT
Physician in Paris

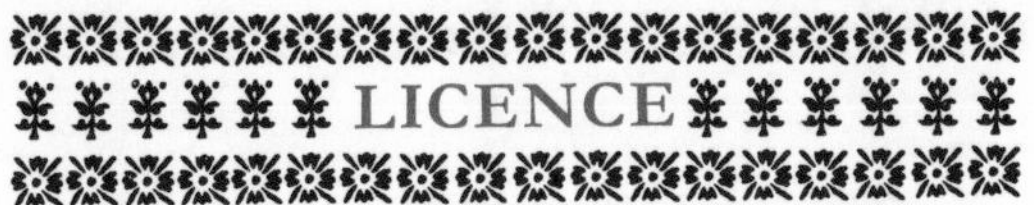

LICENCE

I, the undersigned, Councillor of the King, certify that by order of the Chancellor, I have read *La Decade de Médecine* in Latin and French verse. In which book I have found a practice founded on sound principles and conformant to the best received of rules in Medicine. This is the witness I am required to supply to the public. Given at Paris, this 17th of January, 1691.

Signed, Bourdelot

Extract from the Royal Licence

By the grace and approval of the King, given at Versailles, the 5th of February 1691, signed Dugono: it is permitted to Laurent d'Houry, bookseller, to have printed a book entitled *La Décade de Médecine, ou Le Médecin des Riches et des Pauvres* over a period of six years, counting from the day the printing is completed.

All printers, booksellers and others are forbidden to counterfeit the said book, neither may they sell it by printing abroad or otherwise, subject to a penalty of three thousand livres, etc. Registered in the records of the Society of Printers and Booksellers of Paris, the 25th of February 1691.

Signed, P. Außoüyn, Syndic

First printing completed the 8th of May 1694

The Author Unravels His Argument and Invites the Reader to Study His Work

Let the soldier fight and strut the earth, Greeks, Germans, French and Spanish warriors. Let those who love only carnage and honour exalt the terrors of combat. For myself, I have no love for shields or arrows, trumpets or bugles, muskets or fuses. Peace is what I desire, and that Art so cunning that it restores the moribund to life. Wherefore I undertake this didactic task, which both depicts and allays affliction, which diverts our most distressing days and rouses us from languidness to vigour. You, then, who wish to live in health, read thou my book and long enjoy this life in health.

Nos genus erectum, Christi nos sacra propago
Linquamus veterum turpis more patrum

DEDICATION TO JESUS CHRIST

Son of the Eternal Father, who came for our sake from Heaven, who revealed yourself a God by your glorious deeds, restoring hearing to the deaf and sight to the blind and resurrecting the dead at your coming. You, subduing Death, the World and Hell, saved the slaves and made them triumph. What ardour, what love for us You showed! Away with the proud, the witless, who desires not to know you and does not deign to offer you his finest possessions, his honours, his gifts beyond the tomb. Ah, in Your eyes, O God, Sovereign of the world, our goods on land and sea are as nothing. But Your goodness, Lord, asks us not for rich presents but meek hearts, rejoicing in Your divine goodness. I dedicate today all that Medicine I have acquired over the years and have now composed in verse. Great God, accept it now and let this work serve against all ills and last from age to age. And for my labours, let me taste in Heaven, with the Blessed, a sweetness beyond all rancour.

THE DECADE OF MEDICINE

OR

The Physician of the Rich and the Poor

in which all the Signs, Causes and Remedies of Diseases Are Clearly Expounded

Composed in Latin verse by

FRANÇOIS DU PORT

Physician in Paris

Deus nobis hac otia fecit

PARIS

At Laurent d'Houry,
Rue St. Jacques, by the Fontaine St. Severin,
at the Sign of the Saint Esprit

MDCXCIV

---

and loss of sleep, the loins are heavy. Jaundice may set in, but this is not severe and barely harmful by the seventh day. The palate and the throat feel rough so that one cannot swallow, and there is a bad taste in the mouth and oppressive sweat. The bowel flow is hindered, there is shivering and breathlessness. The varied movements of the bile and of hot fire and vapour devour the body.

CHAPTER XIII

The Signs and Causes of Subsiding Fever

As the fever subsides the great heat ceases, the pulse becomes more mild and little is now oppressive, and Nature overcomes the distressful symptoms so that the patient now appears more vigorous: and thus it is that it is rare to die when the fever is falling, and should death ensue, it is due to some other ill or, because of maltreatment during the recovery, the vital faculty succumbs and perishes. But the decline of the disease occurs when a great part of the peccant matter is discharged by the bowel: and what is left afterwards of urine and of sweat is easily digested by reinvigorated Nature.

CHAPTER XIV

The Signs and Causes of a Benign Illness

When the sickness abates, and there are hopeful signs that the end of the disease is soon in sight, especially if the patient has his legs quite well stretched out between the sheets, and if he lies comfortably on either side, if it causes him no harm to be touched: and if he is quietly awake by day and effortlessly asleep at night, and while awake without distress or delirium: and if there is no fever or any thirst, and he spits well and the breathlessness has gone, if his mind is aright and if he sneezes and has appetite: and if he bears his ill, harsh or benign, complacently, and if his pulse is sound and his complexion that of health: if there is equal warmth throughout the body and if the tepid sweat, diffused, dissolves the ardour of the fever or the disease. If his flanks are soft and no pain there, his stomach emptied and his belly flat, and if he casts out phlegm and bile in his vomit: and if the urine is sound and its sediments are white and uniform and equal, and if the stools pass comfortably from within the bowel and are soft and formed and yellow: then there is nought here that Nature cannot overcome. The cause is a vigorous nature and the temperament that goes with it, but the ill humour comes easy to the coction.

CHAPTER XV

The Signs and Causes of a Dangerous Disease

The disease is grave when it parches and fire consumes within, and yet the outside is freezing: if he lose flesh of a sudden and must stand to breathe: if he spits pus, if he is too wakeful or weighed down with sleep, has vomiting or gasping and the eyes are red, if sleep is marked by fear and trembling and profuse sweating and he lies on his back with arms and legs outstretched: if, with vocal plaint, a lugubrious voice heralds his pain continually like a man hard pressed, if he has distended flanks but does not go to stool: or if, the ill redoubling, his mind is troubled, if all the belly is cold but head and hands are hot: if, despite himself, he weeps as the cruel fever agitatedly mounts from hour to hour, if breathing is fast and forceful and all he vomits is of a piece: if his urine is pale and the brain, now burning, is seized with frenzy: or if the sediment is like scurf or threads, or if, during the fever, there is violent diarrhoea: then these symptoms can only be of terrible import. For they prove that a humour without mercy or an excess of heat attacks all parts and organs and, unless soon counteracted, will lead to early death.

CHAPTER XVI

The Signs and Causes of a Long Illness

The illness will be very long if not too damaging, and the signs are these. If the body is now hot, now cold and the fever brings on sweat, and if the colour is now one thing and then another and there is not too much wasting: and if the urine poured in bottles is pure and the sediment is white and turns red in the vessel or, if already red, is then made white by phlegm: then divers humours in the body have these effects and they will long endure before being cured by Nature and by Apollo's art.

CHAPTER XVII

The Signs and Causes of Impending Crisis

The night before the crisis is always harsh, with pains in the neck, the stomach and the head: with coma, breathlessness, the unwilled flow of tears, and dullness of the senses, and glittering visions and ringing in the ears and quivering of the lips and retention of the urine. Now the attack, redoubling in vigour, presages the crisis, terrifies the patient: he starts and lies awake, mind wandering, he is thirsty, gasps and cries. Nor has he any hope of health, although the doctor – when he has seen before the rigor the sputum, urine and stools confected in good state – knows that hence forward such a patient has the strength to discard the disease. But this great process derives solely from the two great heats, of which the one that is foreign retains these impure humours while the native heat is expelled without, either in the blood that sometimes streams from the nose, or in the faeces through the anal aperture, or from the kidneys or in the skin softened with much sweat.

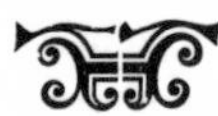

CHAPTER XVIII

The Signs of a Bad Crisis

True it is, these signs may come unheralded, when purging by the bowel is inadequate and the chest expels but little sputum and the water from the kidneys is foul, thick or black at first: and if the dying body loses its vital force, then the crisis is suddenly full of danger. And nothing good can come of this when the disease destroys the strength, and if the humour is cruel and the bile is green, causing dejection, or shows pallor excessive redness: livid, fatty, sticky, black, foaming with blood. And if the kidneys poorly expel the urine, which is foul and scant, strong-smelling and dark: and the sputum full and raging in the throat and not readily expelled, and foaming white while the ills flourish. And the pallid, black and yellow disorders are wholly attributable to the bile.

CHAPTER XIX

The Signs and Causes of a Favourable Crisis

The crisis is certain on the critical day and does no harm if the patient is strong and digestion excellent. The struggle goes better and the humours are gentle and, if well digested, cause less disturbance. The urine is yellow, golden in appearance, and leaves a deposit that is light and white. The soft stools from the bowel cohere, are dun and not at all malodorous: and the sputum is thick with phlegm and bile. Hence Nature's power ultimately triumphs.

CHAPTER XX

The Signs and Causes of Death

When the disease is fatal, the eyes are sunken, the ears cold and their tips turned over, the nose is sharp, each temple flattened and the skin of the forehead hard and dry and taut. The complexion, whether once pale or ruddy, turns blackish: the eye shuns light, tears unintended flow, its blood-vessels are livid black and swollen, its angles gummy, and poor closure of the lids reveals the white of the eye in sleep. The lips hang free, are stiff and cold, the mouth is always open during sleep and he sees nothing with the eye, hears not with the ear, and exudes a cold and stinking lethal sweat. The cold feet dangle, the neck is stiff when the fever is grave, nor will it bend: breathlessness oppresses, it is hard to swallow, he can not devour his food. His words are frantic and he has rigor: nor is it any less horrible that the hands and feet are cold and bare, the ulcer dry and livid, and that the last expiring breath stirs the dry bedstraw, while pain travels from the hips to the internal organs. Extinction of the native heat is the sole cause of death, whether from old age or long fever or debility, or because the body has lacked nutriment, or has suffered too much to gently languish: and hence marasmus comes and wasting follows, or sudden suffocation. Thus there is severe apoplexy, or throttling angina, or the sword provokes an ample flow of blood. And the pain is dire, as when the tetanus crushes the body and mangles it as if torn apart by four horses. The native warmth is expelled by the greater fever that invades and scorches the body and devours all in its flame.

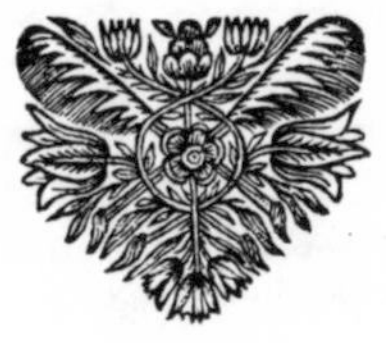

BOOK TWO

CHAPTER I

The Signs and Causes of Affections of the Head in General

When the pain bites an acrid vapour abounds, evidence of an excessive heavy humour. Throbbing indicates heat and, if tension is severe, it lodges in the membranes where sensation is situated and is the cause of pain. If brief and mild, it is due to the fumes of wine, the sun's descending rays, to wakefulness or work: these are the external causes of headache. And if it is long and severe, so much so that it is not possible to bear the sound of voices or other clatter or smells or bright light, in short, all those things that harass the head with torment, then it is the headache properly so-called.

CHAPTER II

The Signs and Causes of the Frenzy

One who is in frenzy has fever with delirium, is panting and oppressed, and this made plain or predictable by loss of sleep, and this disturbed by diverse apparitions. And one of the surest heralds of this ill is that the voice becomes less gentle, wild and harsh, and he is bleary-eyed with a flow of bitter tears, and the vessels of the eye are swollen. He is garrulous, blood flows from his nose, his tongue is dry and rough, he drinks but little, yawns, plucks at his mattress: his pulse is frequent, hard and fast: the urine is palest white, he breathes but rarely, and the fiery bile rebelliously inflames and distends both the meninges and the brain.

CHAPTER III

The Signs and Causes of Lethargy

He is made lethargic whose brain is filled with corrupted phlegm. He breathes but seldom, in great gasps, and his complexion is livid, his pulse wavers, there is tremor of the hands and the urine is as thick as that of pack-horses. His mouth is agape, the fever slow and sleep profound: and his ill is so great that he forgets his own name and all he has learned in life: and this is the main sign that readily indicates this ailment.

CHAPTER IV

The Signs and Causes of the Drowsy After-Effects of Lethargy

When there is no fever in the body, there is sleep and lack of sense or movement, the eyes are closed as if there were no vision: but, inert as is the body, yet the breathing is easy. And when there is catalepsy, though the eyes are open, one remains immobile, insentient, whether sitting or standing. This weakness of the flesh comes from phlegm that is not decayed, and the coma vigil from phlegm and bile together: but the drowsy coma is engendered by pure phlegm alone.

CHAPTER V

The Signs and Causes of Apoplexy

A narrow and short neck is ominous, a heavy slothful body, and vexatious heavy sleep and vertigo: these are the signs that apoplexy is to be feared. And when it strikes, motion and sense fail suddenly, there is breathlessness and severe stertor takes hold: and cure is not possible unless weakness is extreme, and often it is followed by paralysis of the limbs. This is caused by a foul, cold and viscid humour filling the ventricles of the brain, and obstructing the exits of the nerves by which the soul brings vigour to the parts: and excess of blood is sometimes the source whence the apoplexy derives.

CHAPTER VI

The Signs and Causes of Paralysis

A limb that is paralysed has no sense or motion, it is flaccid, loose and heavy, numbed with cold: raised in the air it falls, and if the ill is of long standing this limb becomes stringy, wasted, withered. To sleep while cool by day, or when the shining moon appears, damp or an obstructive cold and sluggish humour, all cause this, so that the animal spirits no longer flow, exert no influence and the movement of the part is annulled.

CHAPTER VII

The Signs and Causes of the Vertigo

Waves, bowling a hoop, running and all circular movement are possible causes of the vertigo. The proximate cause is a warm and tenuous vapour which so acts on the brain and senses that one is seized with vertigo and collapses unless falling is prevented by a wall or other nearby body. And it is considered to originate in the brain when the vision is dimmed, the hearing impaired, the ears have tinnitus, smell and taste are defective, headache oppressive and the mind overcome with drowsiness. But the disorder arises from the lower parts if there is nausea and stomach-ache and distaste for any food that is served: and the patient complains that everything seems to be going round.

CHAPTER VIII

The Signs and Causes of Epilepsy

The premonitory signs of this disorder are many: drowsiness of mind and sense, unsettled sleep, grim and heavy headache, pallor of face and mouth. The stomach is griped with pain and the urge to vomit, lightness of spirit is flown, and vagrant clouds surround the blinking eyes. And the illness now is such that one collapses in spasm without sense of sight or hearing, snoring and shouting, discharging both urine and semen, the limbs are agitated, there is strident argument. It is paroxysmal phlegm that causes this, filling the ventricles of the brain, inhibiting the vigour of the soul to become its torturer: a subtle, cruel, indignant humour which combats and agitates the brain, entering and leaving it, which causes the epilepsy.

CHAPTER IX

The Signs and Causes of Incubus, or Nightmare

The mind and senses are blunted, and breathing hampered, and the voice parched and awkward when the incubus takes hold. The humour that causes this swells around the heart, and the phlegm produced by excess of food and drink exhales a foul vapour that tautens the diaphragm, blocks up the passages of the lungs, and cloudily compels the brain and disturbs the mind with quivering images.

CHAPTER X

The Signs and Causes of Melancholic Illness

There are certain physical signs that make it clear whence comes the black humour natural to man. There is redness and pallor and the skin is rough and dry, with the black vitiligo, and there is wasting. But the two true morbid features of this obscure humour reside within the brain, causing perpetual fear and horror. Then the patient's mind is fixed awry, and his voice utters delirious words. The cause is in the brain, in that it is dry and cold.

CHAPTER XI

The Signs and Causes of Mania

He whose sanity is impaired is full of fury, his eyes glitter and his face is horrible to look upon. His wretched body languishes untended, the whole house resounds with anger, his uproar, din and cries and threatening words are heard afar, his mouth is spread in a rabid grimace: and he adds blows to all these outbreaks, scratches and bites just like an animal. It is not the blood or phlegm that cause this frenzy, but bile that is sometimes yellow, sometimes black.

CHAPTER XII

The Signs and Causes of Catarrh

When the phlegm leads to unhealthy fluid catarrh, cold invades the head, makes the face pale and the voice raucous, there is drowsiness and the urine is foul. The mind is stupid and the senses dulled and the body enthralled by torpor: if the cause lies in the blood, the eyes are reddened and the inside of the mouth is roughened and there is severe headache. There is a foul odour in the nose and the urine is yellow. Sometimes the catarrh affects the shoulders or loins, or may spread to the limbs and inflict countless ills upon the wretched body. The abundant humour in the head provokes the catarrh, which in its turn afflicts the brain and liver, spleen and stomach with air and winds both hot and cold: and the last of these oppresses and the first relaxes. And the same is caused by a damp place, and by food and drink, sadness and roaring rage, anxiety and baneful voluptuousness, until emotion is such as to scorch the very spirit. The cold acts through grief and the heat through rage: but all is resolved if the mind is overcome by joy.

CHAPTER XIII
Of Rheumatism

If, suddenly, an attack of heat or pain affects a limb, it is the rheumatism which is seen to flow down to the parts from above. The humours from the brain, the lung, the spleen and liver flow out and pool remotely, and are especially damaging when they reach a gland or other organ down below.

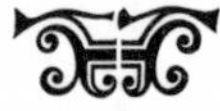

CHAPTER XIV

The Signs and Causes of Ophthalmia

If there is redness of the conjunctive, with tears and matter, and throbbing pain that spreads, this is the ophthalmia: and the cause of this ill is hot blood abounding in the small vessels, which burn and open widely.

CHAPTER XV

Of the Amaurosis, or Gutta Serene

If it is not possible to see, or the eye is less keen, though the pupil is healthy, this is called the gutta serena: and the cause that produces this evident effect is when the optic nerve is totally obstructed.

CHAPTER XVI

The Signs and Causes of Glaucoma and Cataract

Glaucoma is when the crystalline lens thickens, whether due to smoke, a fly, hot vapours, and from this a cloud is installed at the pupil or it becomes thick as a hailstone, what is termed in Latin *suffusion.* This is the true cataract, often called primary, and if the dense opacity persists it fatigues the eye: and if it is the vapour mounting and returning, it will affect both eyes with its obscurity. The false cataract arises from a corrupt belly, and the cause of this is hot vapour of the bile which passes via the brain into the optic nerves, a wandering, deceptive, tyrannic humour: and the subtle humour passing along the nerve becomes established in the pupil and gradually obscures its aperture.

CHAPTER XVII

The Signs and Causes of Inflammation of the Ear

Here there is inflammation in the very depth of the ear, and no swelling is visible, nor fiery redness, but the pain throbs and stings, with heat and fever: and then this ceases once pus is produced. It is hot and pungent blood that causes this, impinging on the eardrum and also on the nerve: and delirium and even death ensue with increase of the inflammation unless it is slight and small.

CHAPTER XVIII

The Signs and Causes of Flatus and Obstruction of the Ear

Flatus without fever, but with heaviness and pain, causes tinnitus, an indication that the meatus is obstructed by thick humour; and the flatus comes from the brain, or from within the body, and wanders to and from in that same part by consent: but the chief air the ear has permanently within itself is always firm and passive. The flatus generates the phlegm and a grosser humour, which blocks the passages and occupies the ear.

CHAPTER XIX

The Signs and Causes of Parotiditis

In true parotiditis there is a red, painful, hot swelling behind the ear: the false is when the swelling is soft, without fever or burning, but that is not true parotiditis. Cold is the cause of this: the humour is long in digestion and the hot humour may cause another and the condition may often be critical, even malign. The head is heavy and drowsiness lays siege, the mind wanders, the patient pants with fever.

CHAPTER XX

The Signs and Causes of Toothache

The torment of toothache is second to no other, settled at the tooth's root or tormenting the nerve or throbbing in the compact substance of the tooth. If the nerve is the source of pain, it is furiously felt throughout the tooth and in its depth, but there is no swelling and the gum is not tender to the touch. The humour sometimes travels to this part from above and, if so, though pressure hurts the pain is not severe, but swelling is either visible or palpable: and the substance of the tooth is inflamed and the heat within oppressive and, unable to find an exit, causes the nerve severe torment flowing from above and inflicting sharp fire on the part.

CHAPTER XXI

The Signs and Causes of Disorders of the Tongue

If the tongue has an unpleasant taste, it is due to corruption by a bitter juice: and salt and acid also foul the tongue so that there is stammering: and the same is caused by abundant humour. But if it is sealed off, and if the humour is dry, it may sometimes resolve: and when it is perverted, taste is denied and speech occluded, there is stammer or a displeasing, thick and grating voice.

CHAPTER XXII

The Signs and Causes of Disorders Affecting the Nose

There is a foul and foetid odour if the nose is the site of an ulcer, due to venereal affection or ozaena: and there is a warm fleshy swelling and coryza. The sense of smell is lost or lessened. The external cause is a wound or blow, from which the ulcer develops with great stink: but often, a salty corrosive humour descending from the head gives stinging pain. If the swelling is hot, it is more plainly due to irritating bile or overabundant flow of blood. Phlegm from the brain begets coryza: and there is a fleshy excrescence that is called sarcoma, which often terminates in putrid ulceration.

CHAPTER XXIII

The Signs and Causes of Inflammation of the Uvula

The swollen uvula often harasses the oesophagus and throat: however, there need be no fear of suffocation. This disorder comes from the gargareon or gurgulio, known as the uvula, and it is distressing and arouses fear that the loose humour may cause suffocation or obstruct the passage of food and drink.

CHAPTER XXIV

The Signs and Causes of the Quinsy

It is difficult to breathe and swallow during the quinsy, and there is complaint of fiery pain in the throat. The cause is a subtle flow of blood that invades the throat and that region of the gullet, starting from the jugulars, and suddenly obstructs the passages so as to threaten to impede the outflow of air and the entry of food and drink.

CHAPTER XXV

The Signs and Causes of Obstruction of the Lung

There is a slow humour lurking obscurely in the depths of the lung, or a crude tuberous swelling or a stone, or a large, dried-up, rounded ball of phlegm: and this is so obstructive that there is severe and frequent cough and difficulty in breathing and unpleasant severe oppressions.

CHAPTER XXVI

The Signs and Causes of Asthma and of the Suffocating Catarrh of Import

If coughing expels nothing from the chest, and breathing is no longer easy in that stertor or sibilance are heard, it is due to asthma, an ill that is without fever and gradual in onset. And it soon becomes a strangling catarrh, and the patient is at times affected by sibilance and stertor, and the breath is oppressed and scarcely drawn even with the head erect. The cause is obstruction of the lung and asthma both: but when a fresh flood of humour follows, you may at once suppose that it is suffocating catarrh.

CHAPTER XXVII

The Signs and Causes of Peripneumonia

In peripneumonia there is dyspnoea and the cheeks are red, the eyes protrude, a weight drags on the chest and breastbone, hypochondrium and back. The expired breath is hot and cough distresses, the sputum is bloody, foamy, tinged with bile, and restless fever is very wearing: the pulse is irregular and soft. But peripneumonia is a double ill: the true one is engendered by a flow of hot blood, but the false is more common and due to a humour of subtler, sharper flow.

CHAPTER XXVIII

The Signs and Causes of Empyema, or Suppuration

Whoever has the empyema feels a heaviness beneath the breast: he coughs uselessly and sweats and his cheeks are red in hue and his eyes sunken: his fingernails are seen to be curved and the fingertips inflamed. And this is accompanied by fever, by pustules erupting round the body, dyspnoea and swollen feet, and by aversion to food and drink. And if his health is endangered, then the sputum is foamy, green or livid pus. A subtle flux from the brain, peripneumonia, pleurisy or the quinsy overflows the mid-space of the chest and is converted into pus and makes the empyema, which must be voided in the sputum within 40 days if the patient is not to waste away.

CHAPTER XXIX

The Signs and Causes of Phthisis, or Wasting

He is hump-backed who is unfortunate enough to have the wasting disease, his ears are withered, his eyes hollow and he is dry with fever, his temples are sunken, his hair falls out, his feet and hands are very warm, he coughs up blood or stinking pus. Breathing is not easy, the ribs are ill-clothed with flesh, he finds his chest oppressed, his complexion is pale or livid, he has swelling. The pulse is weak, the languid body wastes away, the nails curve more and more: and, if diarrhoea is added, it presages death. The phthisis is due to ulceration of the lung: a devouring acrid humour is its cause, a greedy ill devours the tender flesh. He is prone to phthisis who is gripped by slow fever, whose kin are phthisical, is narrow-chested, coughs often but brings up little, has foul pus hidden in his chest.

CHAPTER XXX

The Signs and Causes of True and False Pleurisy

The signs accompanying true pleurisy are these: an acute fever, pricking pain in the side, short and frequent breath, cough with sputum that is often bloody, or at times of another hue: the pulse is small and hard. If it is false pleurisy, it distresses the outer parts, nor is there so much heat, nor acute fever, nor is the sputum bloody or so excessive: the pulse is feebler and less hard, all the signs are certainly less marked, and one can lie comfortably on the sound side. But the other, true pleurisy, is less easily borne: then the patient lies on his back or rather curled up on the other side. The cause of true pleurisy and its severity is effusion of blood into the membrane that sheathes the ribs: and of the other, it is flatus, or a humour, or blood effused into the outer parts of the chest.

CHAPTER XXXI

The Signs and Causes of Haemoptysis, or Spitting of Blood from the Lung or Chest

If frequent cough expels foamy thin red blood, unaccompanied by pain, the lung is responsible. But if the cough is severe, expelling clotted, thick and blackish blood, then there is disease deep within the chest, with a vessel ruptured, opened or eroded.

CHAPTER XXXII

The Signs and Causes of Syncope

If, suddenly, a freezing moisture affects the neck and temples, and mind and senses totter, the extremities are chill, the face pale and there is no pulse or almost none, the enfeebled heart is without force or fire. Various are the causes of this failure: alarm and anger, work, excessive loss of blood or diarrhoea: also grim pain, oppressive and pestiferous air, and insomnia and malignant gossip and fiery ardour, and others besides that dissolve the forces of the spirit and the heart.

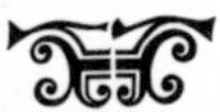

CHAPTER XXXIII

The Special Signs and Causes of Fevers, and First of Ephemeral or Diurnal Fever

Ephemeral fever is due to external causes: the heat of the sun's rays, anxiety, exertion, and apprehension, sleeplessness and anger. But the initial symptoms are not too pressing, for the heat is mild and the sweat a gentle dew, the pulse regular and the urine of its native heat: and the remaining signs are compatible with health, unless the disease ends by altering its nature.

CHAPTER XXXIV

The Signs and Causes of Synochal Fever

This is characterized by drowsiness, redness of urine and complexion: and the pulse in the synochus is strong and rapid, and the predominating heat is mild and dilates the vessels. There is heaviness and dyspnoea is an added burden. There are two fevers, the one straightforward, the other putrid, and the sole cause is an excess of red blood distending the vessels: pure in the one and impure in the other.

CHAPTER XXXV

The Signs and Causes of Quotidian Fever

When the corrupt phlegm attacks the heart, rousing the fire of the quotidian fever, the pulse is sluggish, the body heavy and drowsy.

The cold advances with the fever and the attack is long and the nights severe. The urine is thin and pale and the faeces raw and liquid as they leave the bowel.

CHAPTER XXXVI

The Signs and Causes of Ardent Fever

Among the continuous fevers, however acute they may be, none occurs where the fire is so fierce as in the ardent fever. Whoever has it loses all his appetite, has stomach pains. At first his tongue is yellow, furred, then black, his breathing is far from easy, and were he to cast himself into the rivers Po, Don or Rhone, or swallow down great draughts of water, still he would not appease the thirst that torments him. Ever and again the fever injures and agitates his body, in no way mitigated by slumber. His pulse is hard and the urine, first red, is afterwards quite dark. If the fire descends into the bowel, it does so to no good purpose. His voice sounds hoarse and strident, black blood spills from this nostrils, the clavicles and forehead are bathed in sweat and his filthy skin crawls. His heart thumps, his limbs are dry and hard with cold. His mind is unbalanced and, at the end, convulsions herald death unless the doctor institutes a cure from the first day of the disease. The cause of all this is inflamed bile, excessive work and passion and ill-fame, and impetuous youth and furious rage, and warmed wine and peppers: all of these together.

CHAPTER XXXVII

The Signs and Causes of Tertian Fever

When this fever flourishes, that returns every third dawn, it causes rigor and vomiting, headache and a sharp heat that runs throughout the body, thirst and laboured breathing. The eyes can not close at night, the golden sparkling urine turns dull yellow, the pulse is once more hard and bounding and the attack ends in a sweat. And the cause of this is that bitter scorching bile that wastes the body with intermittent fever.

CHAPTER XXXVIII

The Signs and Causes of Hemitertian Fever

Shivering plus fever mark the hemitertian fever. The humour causing this is twofold: the phlegm and the fierce bile combined engender that ague which frequently and for long returns and burdens. And when the malady is at its height, it is called the trembling fever.

CHAPTER XXXIX

The Signs and Causes of Quartan Fever

The quartan fever, when it comes, penetrates the depths, beats at the bones with cold, followed by horrid shivering and stridor. The urine thins, the pulse delays to come and beats infrequently and gains in force as the fever mounts. The sweat is scanty, the faeces scybalous, and the attack protracted over many hours. The true quartan is a black and putrid humour, cold and dry, it affects the aged, its site is in the spleen: its favourite time is autumn, the blood is thick and burnt. When the bile turns black, it causes the false quartan in the middle of the summer: it is located in the liver, and sometimes the salty phlegm can also excite this fever.

CHAPTER XL

The Signs and Causes of Slow Fever

The slow fever is placid, without complaint of pain, but the diagnosis is uncertain. The pulse is small, though rapid, and does not maintain an even pace. Vigour fades, and the limbs waste, and there is no desire for food, signs that the ill is incurable. The cause is great obstruction by a putrid humour wasting the organs, attaching itself without remission to the brain, lung or liver, kidney or spleen. But wherever it may reside and come into possession, it will be known by its special signs.

CHAPTER XLI

The Signs and Causes of Hectic Fever

The ephemeral fever that comes from heat and dryness and the slow fever born from corruption of a viscus are the cause of what is called the hectic fever. And if this ill affects the solid parts, the pulse is hard and frequent, weak and small, the temples hollowed, the facies leaden and revolting: but of severe pain there is none. To the touch, the heat at first is gentle, but soon more biting, the urine is covered with an oily scum, the skin is as dry as leather, the belly flat and empty and the body a bag of bones.

CHAPTER XLII

The Signs and Causes of Cardiac or Syncopal Fever

Full strong, the fever attacks the heart: and, it may be supposed, derives its name therefrom in that the heart is struck with violent palpitations. There is a heat centred on the stomach, and the breathing is small and frequent, the face red; there is pain in the region of the heart and vapour trickling on the skin. Whether it is judged cold or warm depends on laying the hand on the nose and mouth: and if the breath that emanates is chill, it conduces to sudden death. The cause is violent heat in the heart that wears and destroys the vital spirit; or a vile and perverse humour that causes a malignant air; food that is corrupt and raw and full of poison: and a pestiferous air, and bitter bile that afflicts the heart and stomach with sharp discomfort.

CHAPTER XLIII

The Signs and Causes of Pestilent Fever

A year when the wind is from the south, with clouds, is the herald of a stygian plague that greatly turns to shivering and lays siege. The pulse is shallow, frequent, fast, small and irregular: there is headache, a sad and heavy feeling: the appearance is various and grim and there is often falling and vomit, thirst, dyspnoea, delirium. The patient is cold outside but burns within with heat, and sleep is joined with devouring fever: however do not place reliance on the fever. Instead, when swelling pricks in the groins, the ears, and attacks the armpits like burning anthrax, fly if you are fearful: or, if you wish to cure by Art, invoke God first to ward off that heat which justly, in anger, punishes us guilty mortals.

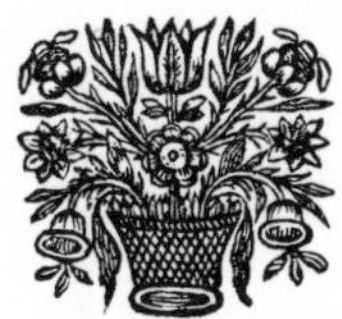

BOOK THREE

CHAPTER I

The Signs and Causes of Diseases of the Oesophagus, or Gullet, and of the Stomach

Excessive appetite and so-called wolfish greed, pica, heartache, the passages too constricted for food and drink, and thirst; all these afflict the patient with a narrow gullet. He is hot and therefore dry and thirsty, thereof is cold and has a voracious appetite: it is an impure juice that corrupts with pica, and excess of humour causes anorexia. The heart is afflicted by the pungent vapour coming from the bile: rarely, it hardens the oesophagus and the stomach is oppressed: or there is a swelling, hot and red, or a foul ulcer. And, if this happens, there is pain in the back and swallowing is irksome, for when the passage is narrowed it is difficult to drink or swallow.

CHAPTER II

The Signs and Causes of a Distempered Stomach

Long-lasting thirst, the ability to drink the coldest broth and make it healthy, yearning to be refreshed within and without, to be distressed by the effects of all hot food, to have nausea, hiccup and a bitter taste: all indicate the presence in the stomach of a foreign heat. The cause of this is exuberant yellow bile, or oppressive heat on the skin, or a salty humour: but when there is cold the contrary signs apply, there is no thirst and hot food and drink are acceptable. Warm poulticing encourages belching. Fine dishes engender acidity and delay digestion. Feelings of cold, a heavy burdened stomach, shivering: these are what inadequate innate heat or the phlegm produce. And if the stomach is overly moist, then too much food and drink and fluid are harmful and cause languor: dry solids are more welcome and much greenish fluid fills the mouth that is not coughed up. But the accompanying bile and also the heat dry up the skin so that drinks and moist foods are preferred.

CHAPTER III

The Signs and Causes of Cholera

The fierce bile presses strongly on the bowels and stomach, and the sudden outburst of vomiting and diarrhoea in cholera herald impending death: for the pulse retreats within and is roused to rapidity: there is gasping, thirst, the limbs are cold and torpid, there is an ill sweat, the nails are ghastly pale: the hands and legs convulse, the reason totters, and death ensues with direst pain.

CHAPTER IV

The Signs and Causes of Obstruction of the Liver

When there is obstruction of the liver, the lower part of the right side is heavy and distended, attacked by pain and stupor, but without fever or any sign of swelling. The prevailing cause is phlegm descending from the brain, which, via the stomach, invades the veins that conduct the aliment and makes the nearby liver viscous: and the liver is slowly obstructed by excess of this thick juice: and the occluded bile, imprisoned in its passage, becoming thicker and more viscid, brings about long-lasting ills.

CHAPTER V

The Signs and Causes of Phlegmon of the Liver

If the inflamed liver is heavy and swollen, oppressed by pain that travels from the right side of the ribs to around the throat, and there is a dry cough, dyspnoea, acute fever, nausea, distaste for food, avid thirst, a furred tongue coated with chronic matter, and the bile is mixed with vomit or discharged below, and reddish urine flows from the bladder, this is engendered by great tumult and flow of hot blood invading the vessels of the liver, where it putrefies and burns and wastes its substance with disease.

CHAPTER VI

The Signs and Causes of Abscess of the Liver

When the liver is sundered by bitter blood and its substance softened, an abscess develops and foul pus is discharged: it is menacing, there is ague and sharp and burning heat and fever, but these subside when the pus appears: and the matter that leaves the part emerges reddish from the bowel or as pus mixed with the urine. The complexion is no longer florid and the body is hot and wasted. The heart, the fount of blood, is feeble, poisoned in its flow, and therefore vigour languishes and the pulse is often intermittent, fast, and weak and small: and the ulcerated liver, whose strong odour permeates all parts, declines all aliment.

CHAPTER VII

The Signs and Causes of Cirrhosis of the Liver

If there arise obstruction of the liver and a warm swelling, this is the cirrhosis: and if this is the true form of the disease, the swelling is hardly painful, nor is there any feeling: and who has this is restricted in his posture and behaviour, for he can readily recline on his right side but is unable to sleep on his left: and the stomach feels as if burdened by an oppressive mass which comes near to suffocation.

CHAPTER VIII
The Signs and Causes of Weakness of the Liver

The weakness of the liver is easy to recognize if a white or crude humour emerges from the bowel, or fluid, or else some other humour like a red issue or blackish blood. And this is caused by weakness of the organ and intemperance, which weaken the patient: and if the attractive faculty is very feeble, a white fluid is passed by the bowel: and if the power of retention is weak, thin pus is mixed with blood: but if the power to form blood is debilitated, what is passed is crude, whence first the feet and then the remainder of the body become all swollen.

CHAPTER IX
The Signs and Causes of Swelling and Cirrhosis of the Spleen

The spleen is often the seat of a soft swelling, marked by dyspnoea and minor cardiac ills: the face is pale and digestion is awry, and sleep is disturbed by nightmares: there is panic, and the left side of the body rumbles with flatulence, and the body is heavy and inert. And the cause of this is sometimes phlegm, or some raw liquor or the frequent use of cold drinks and fruits and herbs. This is what makes the sombre humour:

the lees of wine and limes with blood-red juice. And if the blood abounds and is shut up in the spleen, it is not hurried to the stomach nor brought out at the bowel: it distends, and first makes a soft swelling, and when this thickens it makes the scirrhous spleen which is less painful but more heavy.

CHAPTER X
The Signs and Causes of Melancholic Hypochondria

Sometimes there burns within the body an attacking invading humour, filling the mind with heat and fear, which, when it is fierce, by hard breathing fills up the hypochondria resonantly with wind. The heart falters, beats strongly, then halts suddenly: the face is of purple hue, raging anger is roused, a dark vapour clouds the eyes and these vagaries may cause despair of life. This distemper of morbid obstruction comes when the vessels of the mesentery are filled with malignant humour which the heated liver corrupts, as does the fire of the spleen: and the black fumes fill the brain: and the rumbling hypochondria resound so much as barely to admit of any healing, unless by skilful use of potent herbs.

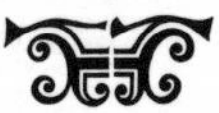

CHAPTER XI

The Signs and Causes of Diseases of the Mesentery, and Particularly of Its Inflammation

Many ills lurk within the mesentery, but the early signs are but trivial and tend to be neglected: because the swelling is internal, it is often deceptive, nor is there really any pain, or fever, or much thirst: but the belly is heavily burdened and red matter and pus are discharged by the bowel. And, as the mesentery is without pain or sensation, no serious symptoms are noticed: and, as it remains a long-term receptacle for filth without suffering from this distressing accumulation, this is the source of diarrhoea and slow irregular fevers, and many other ills whose cause is hidden and unsuspected if the part is resistant.

CHAPTER XII

The Signs and Causes of Yellow and Black Jaundice

Eyes of a green or yellow colour, a flow of bile in the urine, white excrement the colour of the food that is taken: all these are counted evidence of the jaundice, engendered by infarction of the liver, scirrhus or inflammation: or else the gallbladder contains thick bile, not readily excreted, or else a stone or tumour which the bladder is unable to pass. Or the bile, in the crisis of high fevers, traverses the pores of the skin:

or dire poison is drunk, like the venom discharged from the teeth of vipers. Sometimes the jaundice is black, the skin dry and dark in hue: there is fear and oppression, distress in sleep and melancholy by day: this is a black humour that is caught up in the vessels, not excepting the spleen.

CHAPTER XIII

The Signs and Causes of Atrophy and Cachexia

When an organ or other part is corrupted by heat almost to destruction, the body gradually withers and languishes. In cachexia, on the other hand, one is troubled by great swelling and the limbs are heavy and lack vigour. The complexion is pale and livid, breathing infrequent, there is loss of appetite and the bowel's discharge is impure. The stomach is swollen with corrupt humour and with the victuals. The cause of this is a distempered organ in which weakness and crudity develop, depriving the parts of blood and nourishment and altering the habit of the body.

CHAPTER XIV

The Signs and Causes of Hydrops

The hydrops is announced by a poor colour and great swelling, thirst, dyspnoea and distaste for food, and by turgid swelling at various sites. If then the belly fills between the flanks, and feet and scrotum too, and all the rest is wasted, this is reckoned the ascites: and it is the anasarca when there is swelling of the arms and breast and neck and face, and the belly is pendulous. And if the belly swells so as to be resonant and hollow to percussion, it is the tympanites, known as the dry hydrops. The prime cause of all this is cachexia, which obstructs the liver, makes it scirrhous, hot and swollen: and neither spleen nor kidneys expel the black humour, and the gallbladder is full of noxious bile. And if the menses cease and there are not the customary haemorrhoids at the anus to discharge dark blood, the blood ascends and damages the liver, and the true hydrops follows when the liver pours out cool water in place of red blood.

CHAPTER XV

The Signs and Causes Accompanying Retention of the Faeces in the Bowel

A humour fixed in the cavity of the intestines, long stagnant and not advancing in the bowel, injures the ventricle, stomach and brain with its noxious vapour and renders the body heavy and torpid. The cause is a swelling housed in the belly, or a liver burdened with heat, worms or enterocoele, and binding food, such as the quince, and drink: or often an astringent enema, or when the patient is droswy and the senses muffled, or when some other cause makes the nerves replete with humour. The faeces cease when bile no longer traverses the bowel because the gallbladder is obstructed, or when the passage of the phlegm is occluded and, hidden within the bowel, it is rendered chalky.

CHAPTER XVI

The Signs and Causes of Iliac Passion, or Volvulus

When nothing descends from the occluded bowel, the volvulus is the fault: the stomach is turgid and humid and tormented by intense pain with rumblings of wind. Gasping and vomiting and rage and empty belching make their attack, as do dyspnoea, thirst, pallor and syncope, strangury and cold sweat. And finally convulsions herald death and, O horror! there is faecal vomiting. The immediate cause is, as we have said before, retention of the faeces: but primarily, we may suppose, an inflammatory swelling constricting the intestine and wrenching at it like a rope.

CHAPTER XVII

The Signs and Causes of Colic

The patient with distension of the colon suffers nausea and vomiting, and wandering dire colic. The kidneys do not properly expel the urine, nor the bowel the faeces, the belly is resonant with wind that often makes its exit at the mouth. At times, but rarely, inflammation is the cause, engendering vicious bile, and often phlegm, and wind which, by distension, causes bitter colic and frightful pain.

CHAPTER XVIII

The Signs and Causes of Coeliac and Lienteric Disease

A constant muddy whitish bowel flux, but without pain or colic, bespeaks coeliac disease: but in lientery the faeces are not so soft, since the food is not properly digested but, just as it is taken, rapidly translated to the bowel. But the excrement of the former is smooth and bland and liquid. The stomach is weakened by liquid chyle from ill-cooked food, cold drinks or greasy broths or other oily matter, and mushrooms: and so cannot hold its contents. All maleficient victuals, devouring poison, inner disease, damp vapours or the bile can excite these rigours.

CHAPTER XIX

The Signs and Causes of Diarrhoea and Dysentery

If, in the absence of an ulcer, bile or phlegm, alone or mixed together, sink furiously into the bowel, consider this diarrhoea. But if there is colic and an ulcer, and blood flows with the faeces from the bowel, it is dysentery, launched by this bitter humour: but in the former it is less savage.

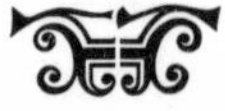

CHAPTER XX

The Signs and Causes of Tenesmus

Tenesmus is marked by a sharp pain at the anus, and urgency to defecate which yields only a little mucus at the orifice, stained with flecks of blood. The cause of this ill is pungent bile, and false phlegm, but more so the adherent sticky phlegm that is passed only with the severest pain.

CHAPTER XXI

The Signs and Causes of Worms

If a devouring worm is hidden in the body, it causes lienteric flux, the belly is racked with rumbling, the vision is blurred with exudate, the face is pale, and there is irregular fever. The nose itches and dry cough is burdensome: and the worms vigorously bite and suck at the intestines: and hence there is tremor, debility and the convulsive disease the ancients called sacred: and this may so greatly afflict infants that they succumb to death. And the cause is not only the crude and putrid humour, but conspicuous fever, without which the earth would not produce and bear the animals it engenders.

CHAPTER XXII

The Signs and Causes of Weakness of the Kidneys

If no fault is disclosed that besets the kidneys, nor any hot swelling, abscess, gravel or ulcer, yet pain extends to the loins and back and affects this site, and the urine is clear as water or else like impure blood: then the function of the kidney is failing. The kidneys are weakened by the agitation of excessive riding, unaccustomed walking or running, a heavy fall on the loins, contusion and injury in a convulsion, and by drinking water to excess: the cold that contains the humour and the heat that liquefies it, emulgent remedies that conduct urine too briskly to the kidneys, or conditions like an abscess or an ulcer which excite severe pain.

CHAPTER XXIII

The Signs and Causes of Diabetes

The preliminary signs of diabetes are many: white spittle, a dry mouth, heat in the belly, cold entering the bladder, and wasting of the body: and it is accompanied by a mighty and insatiable thirst, so that an immense amount is drunk, though less so when there is no coction of the urine. The body's flesh is transformed into a tenuous liquor. The cause of this is fiery heat that powerfully affects the vigour of the kidneys and its faculty of retention: often a vicious, salty, bitter humour that dries up the substance of the kidneys, scorching with fire. The bite of the serpent Dipsas that furrows the Libyan sand produces this great thirst and frequent drinking, though little urine is passed for it is not profuse in the diabets.

CHAPTER XXIV

The Signs of Inflammation of the Kidneys

A devouring fire in the kidneys, urged on by excess of blood, leads to serious sickness and throbbing pain around the pubes, back and loins, and stiffens the extremities with cold. The thighs feel heavy, micturition is frequent, the dried-up faeces are retained within the bowel, the belly is distended with vomitting and belching, and febrile heat incessantly burns at the body. The proximate cause is in the blood, milked by the vessels into the kidneys. But it is the stone that helps to precipitate this pain, or clotted blood within the hollows of the kidneys, or pus or foul phlegm, obstructing the free flow of urine and hence giving rise to inflammation.

CHAPTER XXV

The Signs and Causes of Abscess of the Kidney

This causes a great feeling of heaviness and feverish rigor, and then blood or pus or fleshy matter is passed in the urine, so that pus settles at the bottom of the vessel, whence follows a large and serious ulcer which, whether old or recent, can hardly heal because the urine incessantly irrigates it and stops it from drying up. This abscess arises only when one has not been bled from the elbow or knee in the first days, or when the humour housed in the kidney has not been properly digested.

CHAPTER XXVI

The Signs and Causes of Nephritis, or Renal Calculus

The main cause of kidney stones is said to occur when the urine is clear as water, precipitating gravel, and not infrequently foul matter mixed with blood is passed, and the kidneys are heavy and burden the adjacent thighs, and the spine is no longer flexible. But there is more than one kind of pain: for while the stone is fixed within the kidney cavity the pain is dull, but it becomes agonizing as soon as it comes into contact with the ureter. Eventually, bile and phlegm are cast up in the vomit and then the fire is less fierce: but during the attack it is bitterly painful to lie on that side. The phlegm, viscid and gross, or some other humour, or desiccating heat: one or other is the cause of the stone: and the stones are variously coloured by the humours, but those within the kidney tend to be red.

CHAPTER XXVII

The Signs and Causes of Stones in the Bladder

If the bladder harbours a stone reckoned to be trivial, the pubic irritation causes frequent rubbing of the penis: but if the pain is severe, it indicates a stone of larger size: it hurts to walk or jump, micturition is frequent and there is repeated desire to defecate. The urine is thicker and more turbid, and its precipitate is thick white slimy pus or mucus. In children, the stone may be due to gluttony, in the old to phlegm: or it may be due to seminal repletion, or excess of fatty food like eels and all fish of that kind, which fill the body with muddy matter, and a sticky glutinous juice.

CHAPTER XXVIII

The Signs and Causes of Inflammation of the Bladder

The inflamed bladder causes tormenting pain which produces burning and redness of the perineum. The fever is acute, the penis is felt strongly erect, the faecal passage is obstructed and the urine is retained. The swollen muscle at the bladder neck gives rise to inflammation derived from the adjacent vessels: and if the diseased bladder long inhabits the body, it turns blazingly into gangrene.

CHAPTER XXIX

The Signs and Causes of Strangury and Dysuria

Stinging serum and poor retention of the bladder engender this disorder, named the strangury: for, insensibly, the urine drips away thanks to the defective power of the bladder. Another cause is a more pungent humour, that is painful, the more so if there is dysuria: and the more the ardour of the urine, the more distemper, swelling, abscess, ulcer, wind.

CHAPTER XXX

The Signs and Causes of Ischuria

In the pair of disorders mentioned above the bitter fluid is not passed properly: still, it flows. Yet, when there is ischuria, it is suppressed: the cause of which is obstruction in the kidneys or bladder neck from inflammatory swelling or sticky pus or thick humour or clotted blood, or fleshy growth or mature stone that overwhelm with torment. The ureter and kidney are both full and distended and heavy, with pain in the loins, but without desire to micturate. The mind wavers, from time to time the dying limbs are seen to tremble, the nerves are stiff with cold.

And if the urine is held up in the kidneys, the bladder is empty: if in the bladder, there is a painful swelling above the pubis: one constantly strives to urinate but the effort is in vain. A catheter withdraws much water from the peccant bladder, though this is not possible if it is the kidneys that are obstructed.

CHAPTER XXXI

The Signs and Causes of Satyriasis, or Priapism

If the penis is sturdily erect, but without desire, tightened in spasm, that remedy must be prepared that quickly succours: for the lower belly swells and the jetting of cold moisture is the end of hope. The cause is loss of spirit through excessive patency of the arterial orifices: there is hardly any pain then, but fainting is soon imminent if the affair is not managed properly. If wind is the cause, with accompanying pain, the penis is distended but the danger is less.

CHAPTER XXXII

The Signs and Causes of True Gonorrhoea

When obscene lust does not produce erection, and there is an extravagant venereal flow without producing semen, but a thin fluid flows as crudely as water: and, beginning at the loins, the whole body wastes and the limbs are languid and heavy: this ill arrives when the vessels that prepare and enclose the sperm are enfeebled: and vigour is lost by tenacious spasm, and frequent coitus, or excessive fluid or thin or acrid sperm, or when the sexual habit has been renounced.

CHAPTER XXXIII

The Signs and Causes of Virulent Gonorrhoea

The former is ancient and arose first in antiquity: but the true disease whose signs we now discuss spared our ancestors to afflict our generation. And it is called gonorrhoea, a disgusting and continuous seminal effusion from furtive sexual congress, and its flow is unfelt. The discharge is pale and white in colour, its odour is very foetid, the penis is taut and urinating brings pain that is fierce and sharp. This trickle through the penis excavates an ulcer: and, if suppressed, the poison tunnels through the perineum and matter pours out that was at first confined within. What engenders this malodorous state is a malign poison in the genital parts, dissolving the heat and strength of those vessels where the sperm is enclosed.

CHAPTER XXXIV

The Signs and Causes of Venereal Disease

This dire plague, known to be of venereal origin, infects anyone at all, and its initial signs are concealed and quite unknown: and the gradually increasing pain exacts its due meed of punishment for fornication. In fact, at first it attacks the hair roots, the beard gradually falls out, and hair no longer adorns the temples. The skin is seen sprinkled with numerous spots: small, and yellow, black or red in colour: and then the pustules become large and crusted and dry, around the head and forehead or on the temple, while the rest of the body is disfigured in various colours. The poison ulcerates the throat and palate, and the genitals are also a site for the disease. And when this ill gains a firm hold on the solid parts, the head hurts and is heavy and the malign vapour spreads to the shoulders, periostia, neckbones, membranes, tendons, ligaments and nerves. And the suffering is greater during the night and beyond all reckoning, and the unsleeping body wastes away; and when all vigour is exhausted, there is a corrupt corpse. The cause of this ill is excess of venery and sinful coitus, which first by flow of humour is changed to pus and then infects all parts, grows like a serpent and dissolves the bones.

BOOK FOUR

CHAPTER I

The Signs and Causes of Fiery Distemper of the Uterus

When the uterus is hot, the heat usually spreads and fires the body, the menses are sure to be irregular, the flow of blood is scant and thin and black, it stings and ulcerates but the associated pain is not severe: and a strange pruritus beguiles the senses, as if a bitter subtle humour were confined beneath the skin. The woman is fired with love: all her imagination is fixed on Venus. The cause is an excess of native heat: the uterus is oppressed with hot blood and seed, and flower of youth, and overly frequent baths, a groaning table, the feet engaged in dance with frequent leaping, and abundant jest and delicate word-play.

CHAPTER II

The Signs and Causes of Cold Distemper of the Uterus

In coldness of the uterus the legs waver and give way, the menses fail, love's ardour is restrained, the os and cervix close, the pubes are numb, the loins chill and inactive, the flow thick and repressed and the limbs lively. There is shivering and rigor, the region of the uterus is heavy and drowsy. The cause is lack of native heat, so that there is poor coction of the humour: the blood-flow is scanty in the vessels and there is much phlegm.

CHAPTER III

The Signs and Causes of Dry or Moist Distemper of the Uterus

When there is excessive dryness, the monthly periods fail, the woman becomes sterile and black juice fills the flanks, there is fear of cancer of the womb: and if there is heat, the sacred fire leads to destruction. But if the uterus is moist, the woman is often troubled by the flow, for the menses are more watery and excessive, and the loins and pubis feel burdened. Care, insomnia, labour, anger, hunger: bile, the black humour, the cold north wind and the sun's powerful heat: all these cause dryness. And the causes of moistness are the phlegm and uncooked food, milk, lettuce, greasy soups and food, and sweet apples, water, indolent slumber: a plague to life.

CHAPTER IV

The Signs and Causes of Unnatural Suppression of the Menses

When the menses are retained by some ill cause, the entire body becomes heavy: and this is felt more keenly in the pubes and the loins, the thighs and forehead. There is fever and shivering, nausea, fainting, vomiting, loss of voice, thirst and loss of appetite, and red swelling of the skin where the sacred fire burns. The urine is turbid and passed drop by drop with pain and difficulty: and the chamber-pot is often seen red or sooty black. And last, the mind wanders from its firm foundation, the abdomen swells, as do the legs and feet, the thickened blood is blocked up in the woman's veins. Clotted blood and fleshy swelling and the slow cold humour, the fat and all that is blocked and choked up in the uterus, care and distress, hunger, excessive flow of blood: all these impair and dry up the blood.

CHAPTER V

The Signs and Causes of Suffocation of the Uterus

This strangles the uterus unless aid comes quickly, for the heavy stomach loathes and despises food, leading to loss and emptiness and vomiting. The besieged heart falters, the breath comes thick and fast, the face is red, one feels one is choking, terror strikes cold, there is lack of impetus to speech, the pulse beats weakly and the women now despairs, resigns herself to death. However, these horrors are not certain signs of death, for pulse and sense return when the murmur of the belly softens and the relaxed uterus allows an even flow of fluid humour. The cause is a cruel vapour from the uterus when seed or menses are suppressed: or any foul and venomous humour entering the vessels and travelling upwards that imparts a tremor to the voice and heart and brain: as does the upward movement of the uterus when it presses hard against the diaphragm.

CHAPTER VI
The Signs and Causes of Pallor in Young Girls

When a girl is pale, or blue or green, she dislikes proper food, is harassed by headache and slow fever, her breathing is oppressed and vision clouded, and often palpitations linked with fainting arouse a fear of death. And this is engendered by immoderate use of oil, and uncooked food, and fruit, and frequent draughts of cold water, or by excess of milk or confections of sweet sugar: or by gulping chalk or eating earth or other strange substances which produce coarse humour that blocks all passages and vessels and loads the stomach. And sometimes the girl may eat what causes the liver excess of noxious heat: like cinnamon and nutmeg, pepper and ginger, aloes and other spices from the Indies: which upset the menses and give rise to various diseases.

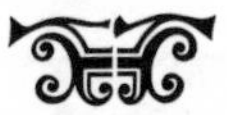

CHAPTER VII

The Signs and Causes of Uterine Passion

When there is uterine passion, salt tears are shed, now unbridled anger, range, now joy: or, like the Maenads, the woman raves of this or that at random and at last falls silent. Nor is she satisfied by Apollo's grove or by Lucina, winged child of Paphos. Venus is in her mouth and occupies her thoughts: an incessant, shameless, secret itch witnesses to her desire for a man. The cause is a vapour from impure female seed which disturbs the uterus, mounts in malignance to the brain, and makes the mind tremble in terror.

CHAPTER VIII

The Signs and Causes of Excessive Menses

Pale is the woman whose menses are excessive: her stomach spurns fresh food, abandons old dishes undigested, however greedily she ingests them: and hence the feet are swollen, and the whole of the pale body, and the limbs are numbed from loss of vital heat. The abundant blood is discharged in excess, nor is it retained by any of Nature's laws but floods out through widely patent vessels, for a subtle stinging heat gnaws within the vessels or causes their rupture.

CHAPTER IX

The Signs and Causes of White Discharge in Women, and Its Difference from the Menses

The bleeding that the passage of the menses excites from the uterus, or from its lining, is coloured red or purple: but the flux, when it is foul matter, is irregular and pale, or yellow, though mixed with blood, and corrodes the part it flows through to create an ulcer whose odour offends the nostrils. And sometimes it is like whey, or issues from the uterus white as cream. An abundance of thin blood and patent vessels promote the red menses: but poor condition and an evil humour, in uterus and viscera, cause this flux.

CHAPTER X

The Signs and Causes of Uterine Debility

When the uterus is enfeebled, the menses flow black or watery and are irregular, and there is no desire for love. The woman shrinks from contact with a man, and if she happens to receive the male semen it cannot be retained: or the child, if one is conceived, appears before its time, or while the periods continue: and pubes and thighs are heavy, loins, head and stomach oppressed. Phlegm debilitates the uterus, and also foul liquor and raw food and unripe fruit, cold and continuing distress, and frequent difficult childbirth and repeated miscarriage, and all that diminishes the native heat: all these undo the ligaments of the uterus, and dissolve its vigour.

CHAPTER XI

The Signs and Causes of Inflammation of the Uterus

The swelling of the cervix is caused by fiery blood: it is hard and retracted to the inserted finger and tender to the touch, and the fundus of the uterus is swollen and fierce pain spreads to the belly and the pubes, and the urine delays to flow. The lower back is all afire, nor do the faeces quit the bowel as usual. The groins and hips are heavy and febrile heat carries all kinds of ills from the groins throughout the body. There is headache, delirium, sweat in the lower parts, all kinds of shivering, swelling of the feet and knees: the pulse is firm and small and fainting heralds danger. A burning flow of subtle blood is the reputed cause, rotting within the vessels of the uterus, putting the ravaged body to the torch.

CHAPTER XII

The Signs and Causes of Abscess of the Uterus

When the above signs flourish, and fever and rigor return regularly and often, then foul matter and abscess are close at hand, derived from corrupt blood that turns into pus. And this flows from the body to the uterus, and often finally makes its exit from within its cavity to the outer air through the opening of the cervix: more rarely, upward to the abdomen, or via the bladder or rectum, or from all of these sites.

CHAPTER XIII

The Signs and Causes of a Scirrhous Uterus

The uterus is scirrhous when there is a hard tumour not yielding to the finger, insensitive, devoid of pain: there is pressure in the loins when the woman sits or stands, the private parts are burdened, the body sluggish, feet and legs awkward in their movement. A thick foul humour engenders this tumour.

CHAPTER XIV

A Description of Cancer of the Uterus: Its Signs and Causes

The cancer is an irregular tumour, resistant to the touch, pale in appearance, surrounded by swollen vessels, a dense discharging fleshy mass: sometimes it is accompanied by an ulcer with thin dark or black discharge, whose foul odour spreads malignant poison. And sometimes it devours the tender uterus and lights a fire in the groins: hairy pubis, lower belly and loins are racked with pain. The cancer is engendered by hot confined black bile, which is wont to erode the soft parts, first the uterus and then both breasts.

CHAPTER XV

The Signs and Causes of a Mole

Often a mole is mistaken for a conception: for the menses cease, the flanks are heavily oppressed, the breasts swell and gradually, too, the lower belly, and the thought of food disgusts. But there is some prick of pain and the complexion is flawed and the body wasted: the pelvis is heavy-laden: movement is neither light nor fleeting in this long gestation and the uterus is hard. And a true mole is suspected to be engendered by profuse menses and useless seed: it is a large fleshy shapeless mass without sense or movement, caused because the seed is unwholesome.

CHAPTER XVI

The Signs and Causes of True or Simple Gonorrhoea in Women, and also of Virulent Gonorrhoea

The seminal effusion attacks man and woman alike. When it is simple, a scanty serous or white discharge comes from the uterine cervix, without venereal lust, distress or severe pain or serious odour. But if the poison is associated with ill-fated intercourse, and foul lascivious ardour, it is dirty, white, yellow or green in colour and stings and sears the skin and has a stinking smell, flows incessantly, and is often accompanied by an ulcer. And gonorrheoa affects men too from the same cause.

CHAPTER XVII

The Signs and Causes of Inflation or Tension of the Uterus

The lower belly is stretched and the pubes swollen, and the distended part painful and taut as a drum to touch. When the uterus contains the winds, the woman sometimes feels it expelled abroad from the private parts or uterine cervix, usually with relief. The cause of which is flatus, or foul humour or clotted blood, which chill and gather and constrict the os so as not to allow passage of the wind.

CHAPTER XVIII

The Signs and Causes of Hydrops of the Uterus

Heavily burdened is the womb affected by the hydrops: nor does the finger encounter firm resistance as with the wind, but fluctuant surge and subsidence, and the swelling is soft to the touch. Like the ascites, the cause is a disorder of the spleen or liver which, by hidden pathways, causes much fluid to gather in the womb. The menses are long suppressed, and all their ichor oppresses and distends the uterine cavity and gradually fills up the belly with stagnant fluid.

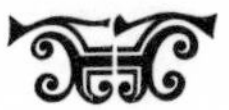

CHAPTER XIX

The Signs and Causes of Ascent and Descent of the Uterus

Ascent causes a painful swelling of the stomach, faintness and lightness of the heart, and tiring breathlessness: descent burdens the anus and pudenda of the woman. The urine is not easily expelled and the woman abhors sexual congress, for the fire burns less fiercely than before. The burdens of repeated pregnancy, a fall or blow or widely spreading humour: all these relax the ligaments, so that the uterus is now at large and may ascend or descend, to get pleasure from those things it most desires or to retreat from what is displeasing. Thus the stomach rejects what is not to its taste and willingly accepts pleasurable food.

CHAPTER XX

The Signs and Causes of Conception

A temor after ardent coitus, retention of the semen and suppression of the menses, the fire of love extinct, the cervix closed, both breasts swollen, swelling of belly, back and loins without defined tumour, the complexion spotty, livid, pale: nausea, debility, loss of appetite, perverted appetite: all these indicate conception. The urine is not trustworthy, nor any of the above signs, unless the foetus is felt to move. A woman conceives when full of juice and conjoined with a man whom lustful Venus favours: especially when the menstrual flow begins or ceases, for then the blood mingles with the seed so that the foetus is formed, takes shape, grows and is nourished.

CHAPTER XXI

The Signs of a Masculine Conception

The woman who carries a male child in her womb is of good complexion, gay and jocose, and, when she rises, is ready to put her right foot forward. The foetus is in that part of the uterus nearest the liver, and there it is felt forcefully and joyfully to move. The right eye is more sparkling: the right breast is more swollen, its nipple erect and dark, it spurts its milk more powerfully and the vessels of the part are swollen with blood. The seed that engenders a male child is hot and potent and fecund: robust and hot from the abundant blood contained in its body.

CHAPTER XXII

The Signs and Causes of a Female Conception

When a woman is pregnant with a girl, she is pale, smiles little, is given to complaint: her belly is more swollen on the left: and on the left the breast also is swollen, but very soft and flaccid, without erection of the nipple, and the milk is easily expressed and watery. Her child moves late and slowly. A girl is engendered by cold seed, in keeping with the feebler female spirit: and as the blood is more chill and moist and crude, the faculties of sense and movement delay in their appearance.

CHAPTER XXIII

The Signs and Causes of Disorders after Conception

When a woman conceives without vicious juices, throughout the time she is pregnant there is no sign of disease: but if she is oppressed with perverse humours, she declines sound aliment but eats rabidly and seeks satisfaction in queer foods; and, unless she is purged or vomits or takes mild remedies, her breathing is poor, she swoons with giddiness, her groins are painful and her thighs burdened, and her legs give way.

CHAPTER XXIV

The Signs and Causes of Threatened Abortion

If the milk flows watery from the breast, and if the infant is dead, the once swollen breasts now wither: the girth of flanks and belly is diminished, the loins and hips are heavy, the foetus does not move as well as usually but turns less often and more slowly. First, matter is shed, all mixed with blood, then actual blood and darkish clots, and at length the foetus is expelled at the same site. Acute fever, gloom and terror, hunger, diarrhoea and flow of blood, quarrelling, jumping and agile horse-riding and running: all these give rise to abortion: and so do offensive perfumes, or a malign odour, or bad or excessive food, and viscous humour: loosening the ligaments of the uterus and filling the cotyledons.

CHAPTER XXV

The Signs and Causes of Death of the Foetus in Utero

If the foetus is dead and retained within the womb, pain affects the eyes and head and heart, and fainting is frequent and the breath foul, there is febrile shivering and the body convulses as in the sacred disease. The lower belly is cold and dependent and cold spreads within so that the cervix is denied contact with the warmth: and because of this the foetus dies and is expelled.

CHAPTER XXVI

The Signs and Causes of Difficult Labour

When parturition is close at hand and abundant blood-stained fluid is shed from the uterus, but there is inability to give birth and labour pains are infrequent and not severe: then it is with difficulty that the child is brought to birth, especially if there is malformation of the womb, the vigour of the uterus is impaired, the passage of the cervix tight and short, and the assembly of the pubic bones too rigid. The stone, or hardness of the containing belly, disease of the foetus, twins or monstrosities, and excessive waters due to firm membranes: or presentation of one or both hands or feet, or of the buttocks or the chest, but not the head, which ought to exit first in propitious birth: all these make labour difficult.

CHAPTER XXVII

The Signs and Causes of Exanthemata

Papules erupt, crowded around the mouth and spreading to the hands and dotting the entire body, with complaint of pain in the head and neck and hoarseness, high complexion, and flow of tears: breathing is not easy, there is itching of the nose and ears and anxious tremor during sleep, and fever and thirst. The cause is a pioson-ous vapour or malignant humour, born of bad air or defective victuals: or of the blood itself or the menstrual flow, producing in due time its manifestations in the skin. And the same occurs to the newborn around the genitals and anus, and children are most attacked, adults or the aged rarely and never in the same way.

CHAPTER XXVIII

The Signs and Causes of Purple Fever

The recent appearance of that bloody comet, which terrified the French and inaugurated civil war and plague, left as its aftermath that ruddy fever called the purple, which, whether old or not, is not mentioned by the ancients, silent on this matter. And its accompanying signs are savage and inconsistent with those of any other disease, for there are both drowsiness and frequent faintness. The urine varies: thus at one time it seems healthy, with no dangerous signs, thin and clear as water: at another, thick, then red and turbid. The pulse quavers and beats often, lacks fullness, is small and usually escapes the palpating hand, not to be counted. The mind wanders and the tongue – most often moist and rarely dry – trembles. The patient cannot lie on either side, but only on his back and that with difficulty. The loins and buttocks and the entire skin are marred with purple spots: the excrement is soft and foul-smelling, ashen, yellow, white or even green or red in colour, ill-formed and almost watery. The patient is hard of hearing, drowsy and his reason discomposed: although, with the disease subsiding, the frenzy remits and he gradually regains his senses as the foul vapour disperses. Perhaps the hands and face are swollen, but if there is no breathlessness one may hope for recovery. This corrupt humour is caused by foul air or vice or excessive food, corrupting the greater part of the blood, whence purple spots are strewn like flowers on the skin: which, if the fever burns more fiercely, assume a reddish-purple or violet colour. But if Heaven sends an air that is more malign, the auspices are bad, the stars more ominous, or the divine wrath has rightly descended to vex us for our faults: then let us first proffer our requests to God and humbly beg His pardon: and only then strive to cure with remedies. Abundant aid. He then will give, the prime source of good health.

CHAPTER XXIX

The Signs and Causes of Gout

If the head is heavy and sluggish and there is drowsiness, and there is a soft white waxlike swelling of the occiput, and the skin overlying the skull is thick and cold and contains a serous humour that descends on the neck and shoulders, elbows, hands, the curve of the back, hips, knees and feet: then the damp head is author of the groaning gout. But if these signs are absent, and the part is immediately painful and swollen, pale or red with but slight fever: then the liver with its swollen blood-vessels is at fault, for the humour sited in the brain and liver is discharged into the joint. And, when phlegm is suspect, the swelling is white and yet there is hardly any pain: but if there is painful throbbing of the part and dilated vessels, and the part is swollen and inflamed, the trouble is in the blood. If the swelling is slight and pale in colour, yet with sharp pains, then yellow bile predominates. But if the colour is dull or black, and the part feels cold and pain penetrates the bones, then the flux that causes this is excited by turgid humour that inflates the joints, or by poisons born of venery or wine or noxious food.

CHAPTER XXX

The Signs and Causes of Elephantiasis

The savagely disfiguring leontiasis known as leprosy or bubbed elephantiasis is ushered in with the mildest signs, with drowsiness and profound slumber: the patient is more lascivious, sometimes his belly tightens as in health, then cold invades the body, the complexion – once so vivid – no longer blooms and the skin becomes yellow, white or black, hard and fissured with open cracks. Later, as the disease worsens, the breath is bad and the voice hoarse, the urine white, cloudy and livid, the face fearfully discoloured and all kinds of disfiguring tumours arise. The lips are thickened and everted to show the darkness of their lower parts: the nostrils are usually encrusted and ulcerated: and the ears are blocked and darkened with a reddish-brown material and seem larger than before: the hairy parts become quite smooth, the eyes are yellow and held fixed, but less brilliant though bulging in the orbits: the forehead is wrinkled in numerous rough furrows, the tongue more or less swollen, both its vessels blackened with the lichen, followed by the scurf and then the leprosy. The patient is harassed by the nightmare, frightened by wild fancies, grief is his constant companion: his shoulders spread like wings over his bowed back, his breathing is slow and his pulse likewise. In the end his body loses sensation and is covered with large white patches. The cause is melancholic blood and all earthy fiery humours, muddy, salty and congealed: often they are black and spread from the spleen or liver to all parts of the body, poisoned and corrupted in all its parts by the malignant force: and so destroyed as to become contagious, spreading the elephantiasis to one's bedfellow through touch, or by the foul air expelled from the mouth. The child born of the seed of one with elephantiasis risks the leprosy, the poison being inherent in the seed: but, so that the young should not be born so much diseased, let them avoid the meat of asses, deer and oxen or other glutinous meat, or food with too coarse residue, or overly heavy wine: and guard against carking care. The woman whose menses are in flood should avoid cohabitation with men, rejecting the sexual act.

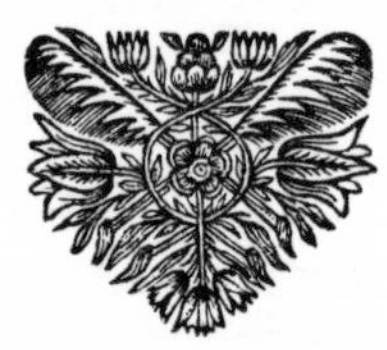

BOOK FIVE

Preface

So far, I have spoken of the body's hidden ills, and said all possible to put them on display, and to relate their causes to their natures were a work of greatest skill: but now I contemplate a greater work to improve the lot of humankind. Sole Son of the Father, by whose Cross Heaven grants salvation, instruct this poet well for without You nought avails. Help me to speak the truth and my physician's hands to heal.

CHAPTER I

The Four Humours
Blood, Bile, Phlegm and Melancholy
Are the Causes Common to Health and Disease

The world's immense fecundity contains four elements: devouring fire, air, water, earth below, from which all forms are made and pass away: and similarly, four humours compose the human body: blood, phlegm and bile both black and yellow. And if it happens that these fashion an even temperament, no harm can come from external fault, nothing is disastrous, but all the senses are pervaded with pleasure and bound up in peace for many years, as told by the Cumaean

Sibyl. But if something other should prevail, such as a putrid humour, a troop of basest ills conflict together and dissipate the native heat: which is so enfeebled that the work is blemished and the onset of old age precipitated, fearful and certain herald of death, which none can evade but medicine can retard, checking the raging humours and restraining their putrescence, and expelling them so that an impure part may not malignantly contaminate what is pure.

CHAPTER II

Every Disease is Expelled by Its Opposite

Etna's heat is nullified by glacial cold, dryness and moisture interact, fire absorbs fluid and renders dry, the thin sunders the thick, hard iron resists what is soft, the rough opposes the smooth, the porous the solid, what is closed or joined is contrary to the open, the sticky to the polished. Thus, lettuce overcomes the bile: calamint and thyme digest and subtilize thick phlegm: sweet almond and ointments soften whatever is rough that they touch: mel roseum removes the slough from a foul ulcer: sticky willow, elm, sanicle and bugle compress an open wound and restrain haemorrhage. Whenever purple humour distends the vessels, opening a vein is helpful: and any residues adherent in the passages are purged by vomitting, urine and sweat, or by the bowel, the nasal openings or the uterus, ridding the body of its humoral content. And if the fire devours and flourishes within the marrow of the bones, a healing draught will cool and water give relief, countering the body's drought: since anything whatever is expelled by its enemy. So that all that penetrates the human body and acts upon it is driven out by an ill that is contrary.

CHAPTER III

Treatment of Plethora

When the vessels abound with florid blood, it can be overcome and thinned by frequent and repeated baths, and much massage, and emptying of the bowel by art or nature: though to reduce it is a Sisyphean labour. But hard work, fasting and copious sweating that opens the pores of the skin, and the belly's flux: all these counter the increased blood and gradually reduce it and protect the body, if it does nothing to cause relapse. And if the illness presses heavily and there is a risk that Nature may succumb, and red oppressive blood do harm, open the veins so that the disease may do no injury.

CHAPTER IV

Remedies that Prepare and Purge Bile

Excess of bile excites many and various dire effects, burning the body with its flame, which lettuce always tames by cooling power, and such green herbs as purslane, hawthorne, plantain, endive and the like, and types of roses, and quickly growing spinach and nightshade found in our gardens purple winter-cherry, inclyta berries and henbane whose flower is white with seed and white bryony, whose juice is blameless, asparagus, sorrel, agrimony, lichen: with violet, water-lily and sleep-inducing poppy, bitter raisins and fruiting red currant, maidenhair, yellow gages, infused seed of psillium, the sebesten plum, prenum, jujube and red cherry, tamarind, vinegar, juice gathered from the pomegranate, yellow pumpkin and water-melon, cucumber and gourd. Purge with cassia, manna and wild rhubarb, and with aloes, kind to the stomach but noxious to the liver: and scammony that occasions direst colic, unfit for children or the old and pregnant: though, for all, electuaries of psillium or syrup of roses are well-known as lenitives, and diaprune that expels all humours: and pills of gold and hyeris and rhubarb.

CHAPTER V

Remedies that Prepare and Purge Melancholy

The remedies that temper the disorder gloomy melancholy creates are bugloss and borage, capers, tamarind, polypodium, dodder, balm that expels care and troubling dreams: and fiery apple valued for its fragrance, cuscata, violet, hop, hart's-tongue, senna, with prunus, whey and sweet raisins: and that herb whose fumes excite tears like those of love, used by Melampus to purge and cure the daughters of Proetus, commonly called the black hellebore, of whose root's rind a drachm, not more, is pounded and cooked in fat broth or taken in barley water, mixed with syrup of violet or mallow, jujube or such like, beaten up together for fear of provoking convulsive ills: and this concoction is known as hamech, a noble liquor full of savour: or else there are pills of Armenian earth or lapis lazuli.

CHAPTER VI

Remedies that Prepare and Purge Phlegm

If the phlegm exerts its force within us, and spreads externally to mar the complexion, then betony and savory, thyme and sage, wormwood, flowers of wild thyme, rosemary, lavender and origanum: calamint and pennyroyal, marjoram, maidenhair, colewort, galingale and hyssop, white and fragrant horehound, mint that is potent to kill worms in the belly, meadow-sweet, parsley, St. John's wort, fennel, scabious, broom, germander, bugle, burnet, camomile with meon, elecampane, the centaury so aptly named after the cloud-borne centaur, and that herb named after Gentius, and the birthwort famed in promoting labour: and roots with power to open and relieve suffering: employ all these. Each warm seed, whether large or small, attenuates thick phlegm, makes it flow faster. Purge from the bowel with agaric, less violently with aloes, and strong turbith agitates all within: and colocynth fiercely plies the body, driving the fluid, thick or thin, into the lower belly. And this is also effected by diaphenicum, mild benedict and diacatharmus, pills of hyeris, light and cocciae, while polychrest expels all fluids.

CHAPTER VII

Remedies to Purge Watery and Serous Humours

If liver and kidneys fail in their natural power, and create water and serum instead of blood, with swelling, then expel these fluids from the bowel with danewort and gentle elder, wild cucumber, cyclamen, and fragrant roses mixing white and red, and those flowers as multicoloured as wondrous Iris in the heavens: and the spurge-flax, not to be taken as a pill all by itself, laurel, ricinus and esula. And spurge and soldanella are powerful too and euphorbia, to be feared and not given to the old for fear of poisoning: and diacatharmus is a purge here, too, and pastilles of hyeris or what the Arabs call alhandal: and juice and tablets of roses serve well, pig's rind or ointment made of spurge, and pills of euphorbia and thymoelea, all are active.

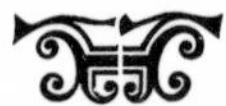

CHAPTER VIII

Remedies to Dispel the Wind

The winds that stray by various paths and rage, shut in the body's cavities, excite dire pains, banished by wild celery and by polium, calamint and galingale: and, if the breath is foul, it is put right by dill, rue and origanum, mint, fennel, aniseed, and the garlic peasants take in place of theriac: ginger, southernwood and cloves and pepper, and that potent poison fennel, carrot, bishopweed and cumin, and fragrant seeds of cardamom, and mustard pungent to the nose and head. And after this purgation, draw out the phlegm with diaphenicicum and suchlike remedies, succour the painful parts with hot fomentations of fragrant mint and thyme: and take tablets of the three kinds of pepper, or aromatics such as nutmeg, spikenard and galingale, and red roses mixed with musk and sugar.

CHAPTER IX

Treatment of Ephemeral or Diurnal Fever

The spirit enclosed within the body's vessels may become inflamed from outward sources and give rise to the ephemeral fever: which, though it may appear mild and trivial, may still excite long-lasting heat, so that its risks are not to be discounted. If it has been brought on by rage, indulge no more in this: if by fear or boredom, make room for gaiety, be bold, intrepid, roguish. For foul excess of wine, order fasting and vomiting and baths; for fasting, eat; for thirst, take draughts of fluid; if work is at fault, prescribe rest: if the skin is too hard, let bathing soften it, and oils like sweet almond or camomile can open up the pores.

CHAPTER X

Treatment of Simple Synochal Fever

Ephemeral fever is often over in a day: but when it lasts beyond this period the ardent spirits burn the purple blood, and then the synochus causes an unparalleled disorder. If this ill occurs without putrescence, it is a simple fever and here is the cure. Let bleeding be profuse, best from the arm, and drink abundantly to cool the body. If then the patient vomits, sweats, has bowel flux or suchlike benefit, these signs are good: yet do not bleed in too close order from foot or arm. If he is a thin man, or weakly stomached, or a child, or one with too much bile, bleed him in stages for fear of weakness or some other risk. In this disorder it is inadvisable to drink cold water if there is the least tumour in any organ, or if there is need to digest a coarse humour, for heat is needed to attenuate this: and it is often known for a draught to give rise to tremor and intolerable asthma. And if one is very strong and vigorous, let him rather be bled until he faints, for fear the blood might stifle him: and if it seems the stomach juices are not acting, give syrup of violets and yellow limes, make broths of poultry and of veal, and a tisane to follow will go down well: and for three days, at night before he sleeps, immerse him in a warm bath to make his body soft.

CHAPTER XI

Treatment of Putrid Synocha

Putrid synocha, because of its putrescence, is uncertain throughout the time it lasts, and the more it increases the greater the danger, for sometimes it contains poison. To overcome it well, begin with an enema, and bleed more than once until the disease yields, making an ample opening in the vein. Purge with whey, senna and rhubarb, uncooked sorrel, tamarind, seeds of lemon, fennel and cardoon. Let frequent broths be cooked with simples at once hot, cardiac and cold: and let verjuice be there and the best meat, like delicately fleshed veal and poultry: and if a roast is desired, take chickens, pheasants, turtle-doves, young hares that live on juniper, and other meats for the sick. Take the sharp juice of yellow lemons, limes and pomegranates: sorrel root and couch-grass infused in water make a grateful drink, nor is it unhelpful to use purest water with pink sugar added. If the vital parts weaken, a restorative cardiac distillate consists of devil's-bit with wood sorrel, herb margaret, and powdered horn of stag or rhinoceros: for such as these serve to deal with disorders of the heart.

CHAPTER XII

Treatment of True Tertian Fever

Tertian fever, which returns every three days, repeating its course during this time, has much in common with the ardent fever, but is rarely seen in our own country or in the Sarmatian lands with their fierce wind: but it is more common in those warm countries where the sun illuminates and heats and burns, like Getulia and barbarous Africa, where raging bile creates vile disorders, stirring and gnawing in the entrails. Let the body be kept moist with meat and drink, the drink be purest water, and give lettuce: serve only meat, making a jelly of mingled flesh of veal, chicken and hare. Let enemas be given and bleed without delay, using a small opening, closed immediately. Induce vomiting and purge the bile: warm water taken with much oil is an emetic. Cassia, manna and rhubarb expel the humour, and cool juices of simples extinguish the heat that burns the marrow, and the primal humour. Then concoct lettuce and purslane, and added to these spinach and endive, lichen, plum and cherry, flowers of violet and water-lily: and mix all these with sugar syrup: and if the heat of the outside air is harmful, maintain coolness with well-water and lettuce, willow, roses, oxycrat. But above all, as we are taught, take care to apply no cold to the hypochondria, loins, thorax, pudenda, feet or any outer part, unless you see evidence of coction of the humour. But when this appears, apply oil like that of roses directly over the liver, use the three sandalwoods, and rub poplar ointment into the forehead, or whatever else may be more useful for sleep: and if the skin be dry, immerse in a warm bath.

CHAPTER XIII

Treatment of True Intermittent Tertian Fever

The ardour of the tertian, that returns every third day, allowing a day's rest between these episodes, is not ill-omened and does not last for long. For the bile that causes this ill is not persistent: and on that day when there is no rigor or burning fever nature can be restored by aliment, a time to open a vein, to relax the belly with a purge and to open the passages of the skin by warm baths: and moist food should be advised. Meat that is suitable is veal, chicken, hare and suckling-pig and pig's trotters: and delicate fresh-water fish and fruit the stomach readily digests: but while the ill persists, vigour is restored by beaten eggs and juice of tisane.

CHAPTER XIV

Treatment of False Tertian Fever

False tertian fever lasts longer and is more frequent and less injurious than the other, and is usually ushered in with a slight rigor: and when it comes one should not feed or purge but take advantage of the quiet periods before and after.

And just as the humour is not a simple single cause of the disorder, so the remedy is neither one nor single: but first expel the bile, and let the food and drink cool down the body, and then further attenuate the tumultuous heat and finally purge down the injurious phlegm. To this end, take maidenhair, lettuce, argrimony, liverwort, senna and violet, cooked seeds of fennel and cardoon, and liquor infused from rhubarb. Such potions best get rid of anger: and added juice of white roses together with diacatharmus more rapidly expel the phlegm. Or first let cassia and diaprune be swallowed, next let a tisane of diaphenicum be drunk if strength there be to drink, then watered wine; and to eat give veal or flesh of kid, capon and mountain birds. If, nevertheless, heat indicates that blood is over-abundant, in summer open a vein on the right side and in winter better lay open the left.

CHAPTER XV

Treatment of Hemitertian Fever

The hemitertian fever is of horrid, fierce and savage nature, excessive to the nerves and harmful to the stomach: and composed, not of one, but of diverse heat and humours, so that unless it cease we see it last for half a year, wasting the body: to prevent which fever remove such filth as phlegm and bile together: but in this period do not purge for fear that trouble follows. But, when this is over, empty the belly with a warm enema and, if necessary, bleed. Purge out the yellow bile, glazed with phlegm, using the remedies for false tertian fever: but this often makes the stomach languid, and you should treat this with cardiacs and sweet-smelling tablets, like rose and ivory, spikenard, saffron, musk and amber, pepper, nutmeg, mace, cinnamon and gemstone, with berberis and aniseed, fennel, aloes, guaiac and coral: take up with sugar and rose-water and give a drachm's weight before meals. Absinth is helpful: and rub with oil of nard.

CHAPTER XVI

Treatment of Quotidian Fever

When the main trouble in the daily fever is phlegm, this must first be overcome, and that by opening the occluded pores: and then one should cut the slow and viscous humour by dint of oft-repeated purging: for this phlegm must be dislodged and plunged into the bowel, which these have power to open: mint and balm and maidenhair and suchlike herbs, making a light sugary decoction to be drunk together with cinnamon and guaiac for a zest. If you wish to cleanse, infuse agaric: and as an antidote take turbith and scammony, for these conduct the phlegm. And, when all is in order, give turtle-doves and partridges to eat, thrushes, quails and partridges: add salt to the bread, or aniseed, ground coriander or such: and do not give water only, but mix with wine. As for opening the swollen vein with the scalpel, activity of the disease forbids this: however, if the fever does not remit and the urine is thick and fiery-red, let the blood jet out but take care that the flow is not too abundant.

CHAPTER XVII

Treatment of Quartan Fever

Do not purge excessively at the onset of the quartan, for to be too zealous in the first attack may hamper expulsion of this coarse humour and so exacerbate it as to cause more distress. An enema will more comfortably do what is necessary, with a lenitive: and then, when matters allow, you may open a vein. For food, give young calf, lamb, kid, capon and fowl and saucy, chattering partridge: the juice of all of which is good to rally the wavering forces of digestion. Then it is right to purge with senna, whey, both joined with bugloss, sclae-fern, fumitory and dodder, tamarind, yellow flowers of broom to infuse the Indian confection popularly known as hamech. Give hot baths to excite sweating, and certainly both theriac and mustard have their place here. But use all of these with caution, not to re-ignite the fever in a dry body: and when the attack of fever is over, hunger appeased and the patient restored by sleep, immerse him in a warm bath.

CHAPTER XVIII

Treatment of Slow Fever

When the region of the belly, liver, brain, lung, kidney or spleen contains a humour followed by slow fever that obstructs their passages, then gradually and often purge their stagnant filth with the proper remedies until the cause of the disease recedes and the true nature of the corrupted part is restored. If the head is affected, purge with agaric: or fortify by adding rhubarb and balm, betony and waterlily, violet and rose: and after food give conserve of roses and preserved seed of fennel or coriander. If the liver is affected, give agrimony and endive infused with senna and rhubarb, which purge and digest all useless humours. But herb margaret gives comfort to the heart and cassia is an antidote for humour in the lungs or kidneys: senna is suitable for the spleen, but add to it capers and tamarind: and resolve troubling wind with bark or aniseed, celery or horehound. Take care, if bleeding creates excessive flow, to quickly bind the wound lest heat may irritate and corrupt an organ and all end in irreparable wasting.

CHAPTER XIX

Treatment of Cardiac or Syncopal Fever

Unless you rapidly relieve the cardiac fever, often accompanied by syncope, the patient may suddenly collapse and die. Therefore apply to the nostrils aqua vitae, rosewater, camphor and vinegar, so that their odour may revive the forces. Let the warm blood flow from a vein, refresh with cool air by gentle agitation of a fan, and with a warm cloth foment the chest with vinegar, rosewater, bugloss and water-lily, together with sandalwood and seeds of hermes oak and saffron. Make a rose ointment with powdered musk and amber, and give to drink the sugared juice of pomegranate or wood sorrel. And restore rapidly by mixing wine with water: let the diet be liquid, adding acid to the flesh of kid, give easily digested broths and jelly of poultry: use powdered horn of unicorn or stag, gemstones or benzoardisc to expel toxins and snake venom from the heart.

CHAPTER XX

Treatment of Consumptive Fever

When a consumptive fever occupies and burns the body, bleeding is fruitless, nor should the belly usually be troubled with a purge. Cold remedies are helpful, and moist juices: therefore use cream of barley and broths of veal and young kid, lettuce and fresh leaves of purslane: give woman's milk or milk of cow or goat or slow-footed ass, or of sweet almond. Express the jelly or distil the broths of snails, of turtle, plump turtle-doves and fowls. Liquorice water relieves thirst and makes a black mixture with white Indian sugar, stoned figs and raisins, jujube and violet syrup. If the stomach languish and the body's forces fail, use but little wine: soften dry skin with sweet water: let the air that enters the nostrils be warm and moist. Sleep is promoted by water-lily and seed of lettuce and white poppy, calm rest and song. Apply a poultice to the heart made of conserve of violets, roses, water-lilies and added vinegar: and often smear the chest with freshest butter, making a pleasing linctus with sugar syrup: and for food give beef-broth. And in this fever the limbs are comforted by cream curdled from milk and freshly expressed cheese and beaten eggs.

CHAPTER XXI

Treatment of Pestilent Fever

The fever that infects the public from the air is wont to lay thousands prostrate in death if diligent care does not afford a cure. However, to overcome it, light a fire in the hearth, purify the entire house with incense: open the windows to the winds from north and east, but not the south for the warm zephyrs harm. Let all be bright and tidy: let the attendant's words and glance encourage, and expel the fear of death. And then, from earths and gemstones, animal and metallic agents, let the physician choose those antidotes that provide an aid to health, like theriac, mithridatum, alchermes, the red zircon, those named after eggs and pearls. Extract the juices of different plants, like scabious, meadow-sweet, balm, wood-sorrel, germander, blessed cardoon:

and chicory, tormentil and rustling juniper, borage and bugloss, thapsia: and you may add to their virtues with draughts containing powder of bezoar, the horn of long-lived stag, or that which grows from the forehead of the unicorn. What is easily digested is the best food: good juices, broths and jellies are useful here: and a distillate fit to restore the forces is cooked flesh of calf, pigeons, turtle-doves, fat thrushes, pullets, capons, partridges and pheasants and other woodland birds, with odorous herb margaret and powdered gemstones. Water is worth more than wine: however, a drop of wine diluted with several drops of water may do some good. The food and drink will be improved by sprinkling with purple pomegranate, and by the juices of fruits like acid limes and yellow lemons and purple red currant and pippins, finest produce of the garden. Let pills be made of aloes, myrrh and saffron if the air causes this ill, but no other purges: but if this affection comes from a putrescent humour, and there is a glint of fire in the face and eye, or breathing is difficult and the throat painful, the urine red and the pulse bounding, if the commencing ill is burdensome: then you can bleed freely and purge with moderation: but if the patient is stronger, let him be purged more vigorously: and purgation done indifferently often succeeds despite mistakes, provided only that the surgeon is cautious.

BOOK SIX

Preface

It is given to man to raise his eyes to Heaven above, and to aim to render himself so worthy: but if, too full of gifts, he aspires to excel and raise his glory to the heavens, there is no part of his body that is immune to torment. Disease attacks at every point, the whole man may be sick, his noblest part brought down in ruin: although his heart be stout, the least shock undermines it, and when he is injured by pestiferous air the heart is the first to be affected. The mind's residence is in the brain, and most often is dislodged by coma or raging frenzy. But the Art of Medicine is a gift from God, who expels the most unkind ills from our bodies. The way that this is done is the subject of my Muse: befriend my soul, O Holy Spirit, without whom all labour is in vain.

CHAPTER I

Remedies Indicated for the Head, Known as Cephalics

To begin, I shall treat of disorders of the head and list those drugs more fitted for the brain, so that the novice may confine himself to those more commonly in use. If, therefore, phlegm oppress the head, try balm, sage, elder, calamint, rosemary, betony and laurel, horehound, and flowers of such fresh herbs as lavender, savory, nigella, euphrasia that clears old persons' eyes, mint, camomile, galingale, melilot, dill, root, seed and flower of seapeony, rue and iris, wild thyme and thyme itself, Indian nard, the lesser centaury: to which musk may be added, and castoreum and nutmeg. To overcome the bile, take violets, roses, lettuce, water-lily, the nightshade common to our gardens that rids the head and ears of pain: and white-seeded henbane, evergreen, the corn poppy, the slow willow, the myrtle linked with Venus, and drowsy mandragora: all extract the juices from the body.

CHAPTER II

Treatment of Headache

Headache is a notably fierce pain, whose cures and causes are various. If simply due to heat, let cool air be breathed, and to drink give a tisane or water only, or mixed with a little wine. Lettuce is best to eat and confers rest and slumber. Smear the forehead over with a cool ointment like rose with poplar: or moisten with the juices of nightshade, houseleek, violet and rose, mandragore or henbane and white poppy: if the humour is hot, opium and vinegar may be added. If the bile rages, give water-lily, senna, violet, juice of white roses, so-called black cassia: these, taken together, cleanse the site: for plethora, open a vein. If the headache has been brought about by cold, give flesh of mountain birds, and bread salted and seasoned with anise, and old wine. Dry heat, work and abundant sleep are moderating. Rub powdered amber and nutmeg into the forehead and oil of laurel and green myrtle. First purge the body: if the disorder is caused by a cold humour, use the agaric fungus that grows on trees: if the disorder is dry, moisture simple and alone causes less disturbance: but when both are harmfully involved a contrary is indicated.

CHAPTER III

Treatment of Cephalea

When the headache is long-standing, various remedies are available: of these try the more moderate, but seek the source of this enduring pain. Sometimes it is due to an extreme heat: if the pain is stinging, expel the bile with rhubarb and manna, and white roses have their use. If it is heavy, then bleed often: and if it is what is called basilic, or from the brain, relieve the pain with violets and white poppy, water-lily and flowers of this kind. But often the cause is a chill vapour, or the winds, or a cold thick humour: therefore frequently administer pills which expel the phlegm from cavities, or give a potion of diacatharmus or diaphenicum mixed with senna, for this alone can clear the brain, keep the body youthful and retard old age, voiding the darkest humours from all parts. Have the head shaved for these protracted pains, rub in with oil of spurge and castoreum, mixed with oxyrhodium. Prescribe sage and mastic, pepper and pyrethrum: as snuff, give juice of pimpernel or cyclamen, or else of marjoram, beet, hellebore and mustard: amber and nutmeg if the subject is delicate: and then also use perfume of mace, incense, varnish and wood of aloes all together: styrax and benzoin as a powder with spikenard and lemon-peel all made with gauze into a nightcap: and construct a pomander with pure ladanum, gum of tragacanth, amber and musk. And if this altogether fails to overcome the ill, bleed from the forehead veins, put cupping-glasses on the temples, puncture the thighs, arms and buttocks: and at last the cautery will have to be employed, even perhaps at sites other than the head.

CHAPTER IV

Treatment of the Frenzy

When the brain is possessed by the raging frenzy, use frequent broths and infused herbs, emollient and cool: like sorrel, purslane, saffron, houseleek, and lettuce that extinguishes love's passion and is unequalled for inducing peaceful sleep. Let veal or flesh of kid be cooked in butter, and give in the anus an enema of whey, and give prunes and those else that gently move. Open the median or cephalic vein if there is plethora: if the disease persist, bleed from the forehead, beneath the ear or below the tongue, and this without delay lest, being wounded, he may wound you, or, by interfering with his wound, may by misfortune so cause the blood to flow as to be author of his own death. Black cassia is superior to rhubarb, is more emollient, expels the bile more gently: however, an infusion useful to be drunk is one of lettuce, endive, violet. Water, not wine, is helpful, boiled to a syrup with sugar and juice of limes, except perhaps a tisane of liquorice mixed with barley. If none of this arrests the frenzy or permits of sleep by night or day, all art must be applied for sleep lest the brain burn up with fire, greedily consumed: therefore admit little light where the frenzied person is, keep him in the dark: scarify the back and draw blood with cupping-glasses and let leeches suck at nose and temples. Anoint the shaven head with oxyrhodium and the forehead with poplar mixed with vinegar: give mandragora juice, nightshade, water-lily, saffron, a little opium: the cream of barley cooked with cold seeds and taken with white sugar at night confers quiet sleep: or else cool syrup of water-lily, violet, poppy and roses. Let either foot be bathed in warm water infused with houseleek and vine-shoots, willow and vernal violets and roses: but betony and camomile and mallow infused foment the brain. And let a chicken, dog, pigeon or other animal be opened while alive and placed on the head to draw out the vapours from the brain and check the contending fire. Bind the patient firmly if he rages to overcome his force and threats: and if his bonds cause heat, so much heat will be drawn from the brain.

CHAPTER V
Treatment of Lethargy

Lethargy induces great apathy and profits nothing: therefore speak out and study what arouses the lethargic's interest: the trumpet's clangour for the soldier, silver and gold to bedazzle the miser quickly expel languor and drowsiness: though these cannot succeed completely unless the cause of the lethargy is overcome. Therefore remove this with a suppository or enema to soundly move the sluggish bile. If necessary, open a vein in the head. Pound the flesh of simple hyeris or bitter colocynth to give as drink: nor is white agaric less useful, macerated in warm betony water with added seeds of ginger. Use thyme, calamint and pennyroyal as snuff: and pour on the shaven head oil of pepper and of laterum: foment the head with origanum and savory, try cupping the neck and back and thighs and loins, using greedy fire. Wine helps, but better still is water infused with sugar or honey: roasts are best to eat, and the whitest bread.

CHAPTER VI

Treatment of the Carus, Catochus or Catalepsy

Soporific carus causes coma, much like lethargy, but the cause of carus is so powerful as to require stimulants and to be attenuated. Make a good draught of hyeris or whatever else expels phlegm from the bowel: vigorously rub and bind the extremities: pull out the hairs from head and beard, do not spare those of the pudenda but avulse those of these parts, rousing from sleep with the sharp sting. Castoreum is useful, dissolved in hydromel or aqua vitae: snuffs may be tried, and hot applications to the shaven coronal suture such as powder of cantharides, pigeon's dung, garlic, cress mixed with seeds of squill. Give honeyed wine, put mustard in the food. The coma vigil of catochus is known as catalepsy: and, if due to purple blood, it is evidenced by a red or livid face and calls for bleeding, but preceded by an enema. If the head is burdened by cold, purge with those invaluable pills called pills of light or gold: or mix hyeris in betony water: rub in oil of iris or of laurel, castoreum, rue or fennel. Use cold remedies if the source of drowsiness or vigil is burning heat.

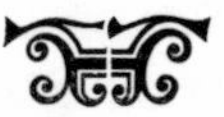

CHAPTER VII

Treatment of Apoplexy

Apoplexy comes on quickly and is soon over and rapidly destroys a man. Apply vigorous friction and compress with bonds: have the patient in a well-lit place: if it is apolipsy, open an elbow vein or release the blood stored in other vessels at the temples, head, back and tongue: and if the flow is too slight, apply cupping-glasses or leeches to the skin. Make a suppository with gem-salt, seeds of rue, honey and powdered hyeris to alert a sluggish bowel: and to the palate apply an infusion of the herb calendula mixed with aqua vitae and castoreum, theriac or hyeris, whose conjoined power is effective. Or give salt and stinging mustard to restore the spirit and cut the cruel humour: hold above the head a red-hot frying-pan; make a soft cap with Vigo plaster for the head. Exhibit fragrant costmary, nard and iris, and attach a blister to the head where the suture is evident. Prescribe nutmeg water and cassia, let him breathe the odour of honeyed wine: when the attack has been dispelled by these measures, vigorously expel the phlegm to avoid recurrence.

CHAPTER VIII

Treatment of Paralysis

If any part is weakened, let it be rubbed with olive oil, but first give an enema: and if copious bleeding is indicated, use the veins of head and tongue. Sweeten the water drunk with sugar and cinnamon, or infuse with hydromel, sugar and iris, for wine alone is bad for the nerves. Roasts are useful food. Sage, marjoram, calendula, the true primula, wild thyme, origanum, laurel, dwarf elder, garden thyme and juniper, boiled together with a fox in water, make a bath to immerse the paralytic: or you can make a fomentation by soaking towels in the hot liquor, and let the vapours given off be absorbed by skin and mouth and nose. And massage the affected limbs with balsam of Peru and other balsams. Roast brain of hare, together with conserve of rosemary and powdered nutmeg, prove useful. Purge with such drugs as senna, turbith and agaric: and a vomit does no harm. The so-called sarsaparilla, macerated with guaiacum in warm water, makes a drink which dislodges the coarse humours of the body and expels sweat through the fine pores of the skin.

CHAPTER IX
Treatment of Vertigo

If turbid vapour, heat-engendered, is the cause of the blind vertigo, relax the bowel with bland enemas: section the median vein if the vessels are distended with blood, and often those that beat behind either ear, and attach cups to legs and back: smear the head with oxyrhodium. Rosewater and pomegranate juice mixed with vinegar, infused with sugar-cane for sweetness, yield a fluid to be drunk without added wine: Bacchus and Venus are best avoided: yet, for the crude vertigo, old wine taken with water to avoid fumes has its uses. Onions, beans, lentils and chickpeas, foods producing wind, are harmful unless joined with dill, hyssop or horehound. Let the food be dry, for dryness is good: roast pigeon, fowl and partridge. A pill to purge the brain and stir the bile and phlegm is useful, also to relieve the burdened stomach, whose windy vapour is often the cause of this disorder: thereto, make a fortifying tablet of rhodium, once the preserve of abbots, and wormwood infused in water, warmed with red wine, and add the three sandalwoods of these.

CHAPTER X

Treatment of Epilepsy

When there is a violent attack of this disease, keep the head upright: rub the jerking lower limbs with a rough towel, separate the teeth by hand or with an instrument, open the mouth by force: remember to mix juice of theriac and rue and apply it to the tongue and soft palate with a feather: or take castoreum dissolved in oxymel, squill, benzoin and pitch and introduce this oil with a feather into the throat to induce vomiting: and instil black hellebore and pyrethrum into the nose. Also, use hyeris and such to purge out the phlegm. Open the popliteal vein, or the great or small saphenous, though the haemorrhoids may be more available. Apply the cautery to the nape of the neck and cup the back, so that the flame may draw forth abundant blood. Release the secret forces of the human brain with seed and root of peony, the mistletoe of oak, the rennet of a hare, the heart of wolf, vulture or mole, the liver of a kite of fox's brain, the stone found in the stomach of swallows or chickens. Testes of boars or swaggering cocks, coral, stag's horn, the hoof of elk and slow-stepping ass: powder these with sugar or mithridatum or rosemary conserve: or use cinnamon or theriac with water, water of guaiacum, china root or sarsaparilla: and the flesh of weasel is a relief in this disease. But do no harm to children at the breast with any of these agents, which may upset the strongest: but gird them with a collar of jasper, peony or green emerald: nor should the wet-nurse indulge in venery or wine, but stick to water, either pure or mixed with honey, and easily digested food. The best diet in this disease is delicate and dry.

CHAPTER XI

Treatment of a Nightmare

To put an end to a nightmare, let light expel the darkness, and let the doctor take care to shake and rouse the patient from slumber, forcibly squeeze and double up his fingers, and with an enema expel downward the cloudy vapours that obstruct the paths of heart and brain. If the body is plethoric, do not hesitate to open a vein:

and purge with pills of hyeris and lapis lazuli, and others grateful to the stomach. Nor will white agaric, hyssop and horehound macerated with senna in warm water do any harm: neither the snuffs prescribed to draw the phlegm along the palate. Apply cupping-glasses to the thighs and shoulders and give paste or powder of gemstones, coral, coriander, red roses, and seed of the black peony. Comb the hair with an ivory comb. And the victuals should be digestible, mead or fine wine: eat little in the evening and take no food whose vapour may obstruct the brain.

CHAPTER XII

Treatment of Melancholic Illness

When the black humour has settled in the brain, expel it with an enema, or gently purge with lenitives like senna and whey, cooked with apples, and seeds of horehound, lemon and bugloss. Open the cephalic or the median vein, or the main cubital if the spleen or liver is the main cause of the disease: and if the periods have stopped, continue purging and open the veins around the ankle. If none of this assuages the disease, for a stronger purge give hyeris, or so-called hamech or diaprune: and, if this too does not work, try hellebore, or the Armenian pill is excellent in power, and lapis lazuli, and certainly the plant called fumitory. Open a vein in the head and obtain sleep by means of violets and lettuce and water-lily flowers. Immerse the patient well in a warm bath: the steam will rejoice his heart. Make a drink from gemstones and chermes mixed, and theriac and bugloss water, or water drunk with wine. The flesh of calf, roebuck or fowl are sound sustenance, available in every country home: and give white bread and water mixed with wine.

CHAPTER XIII
Treatment of Mania

Sometimes the head is filled with raging blood, or black humour, or excess of burning yellow bile: hence this frenzy. First give an enema, that the mind should not be finally overwhelmed and perish from excessive fervour of the blood: then open the median, next the cephalic vein. And then expel the humour with lettuce, tamarind, manna and senna: but this horrid frenzy will always yield to syrup of violet and borage, to which add fumitory and endive: but if these avail nothing, then give cassia, senna, hop and diaprune, made into a syrup with white roses. But rarely renew the opening in the vein, and soften the body often in a tepid bath. The diet used for melancholy serves also for the frenzy: and in the latter one should take but little wine, or none at all, but drink tisane or water boiled with sugar.

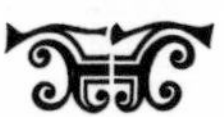

CHAPTER XIV

Treatment of Catarrh

Catarrh is a common affection of the human race, and may be minor or severe: and it is born of piercing cold, or heat. When hot and light, foment the head and sutures with roses in a soft cloth: rub into the forehead ointment of roses and oil of water-lily mixed with a little vinegar. A cooked pear, a quince or coriander will check the fumes of supper: and give rosewater in the evening. But when the body contains much detritus of bad humour, first drain blood from a vein: and then it is proper by purging to extract noxious fluid humours from the bowel by yellow so-called golden pills and diaprune: all serve to relax the belly, as do scammony and rosewater: and after this give a relaxing bath. But if this serves for nought and the continuing bitter flow causes cough and loss of sleep and frequent hiccough and soreness of the throat, exhibit tragacanth and the orange powder of Armenia, or the sigillated earth of Turkey, Sabaean frankincense, amber, oil of spikenard, veronix, camphor, the dry conserve of roses, or syrup made of myrtle with water-lily or poppy: for these in highest degree induce sleep, condense the subtle humour and lessen its aggression. But when the catarrh is cold, and not so troublesome, take enough millet, bran and salt: pound and roast the salt and millet and mix with the cold bran, and fill a little bag and apply this to the head and thus dry thoroughly. And if the phlegm with which the brain is laden threatens sudden collapse, support from below by rapidly relieving the belly via the bowel, using such remedies as senna and agaric, colocynth and turbith. See that the patient spits and blows his nose to rid himself of phlegm: and perfumes are good for this, and you can also use them in a nightcap: apply ligatures to arms and legs like a torturer: and use cupping with red flames and the seton and the cautery that leaves its brand: and yet, these agents are often dubious in value and leave health more uncertain. However, let the midday meal be long, and supper small, and let him sleep sound at night, if not by day: and avoid the sun's rays and the bicorned moon and Aeolus's errant winds.

CHAPTER XV

Treatment of Rheumatism

If the flesh is suddenly beset by pain and burning fiery heat, causing the rheum, insert a suppository or enema by the anus: and then bleed freely from the elbow: purge with the right remedies: and certainly, if the returning fluid contains bile, give manna, rhubarb and juice of white roses. If there is abundant whitish phlegm, expel it with agaric and the usual remedies. Support the part to which the flux has roved and, if this should be the knee, repel with various astringents, such as oxyrhodium or oil of roses with houseleek. It is worth trying barley mixed with flour as a red desiccant, adding calcite. If the pain is very severe, relieve with a poultice of white breadcrumbs mixed with milk, butter and water of roses or of houseleek: and place oxycrat thereon once the pain is worn off and the flow of humour is over.

CHAPTER XVI

Treatment of Ophthalmia

If the coat of the eyeball, called the conjunctiva, is red and inflamed, the juice of plantain and of roses, and white of egg and woman's milk, will take away the pain: but instil these quickly, while the discharge is still not great: but if it is severe, first inject an enema, open the main vein, known as the median, and then the so-called cephalic. Purge first with a bland remedy, such as that called the lenitive, cassia, manna, rhubarb, all that expel into the bowel: and add diaprune, rosewater or diaphenicum if the phlegm abounds. And if the ophthalmia persists for some days, use the so-called golden pills and those-called alephangina, or pills of light or of hyeris: and white agaric, formed in a mass or given as a drink, may not be harmful. And if all these do not undo the heat of the disease, apply the purple flame of cupping-glasses to the shoulders and repeat, and leeches to suck around the eye: open the veins that throb on forehead and temple. Use Rhazes' eyewash and a poultice for the forehead made of myrrh with incense and flour at will, with white of egg as the excipient. And, if all this fails, the cautery applied to the front or back of the head restores health. Baths are no use in the first days of the disease, but towards its end relieve the pains.

CHAPTER XVII

Treatment of Suffusion, or Cataract

When the cataract arises from the stomach, relieve with pills made of hyeris: but the other form, which is due to disorder of the brain, if susceptible to art, is treated by coccia pills to dislodge the phlegm in rue and fennel water. Prepare an eye lotion with juice of calendula and honey and gall of goat, sheep, cock, hawk or crane. The fluid distilled from honey, whether pink or ordinary, is potent, but that made from squill is stronger and the sagapenum should be duly tried, dissolved either in that water, or in infant's urine or in fennel water: and use balsam or pounded bone of cuttlefish or white sugar. Apply massage often to the head, ligatures to the limbs, and cups to the neck to secure good flow of blood, and black caustic to the coronal suture. If the humour remains obdurate and does not yield with time, let an oculist remove it from the body.

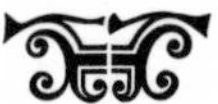

CHAPTER XVIII

Treatment of Amaurosis, or Gutta Serena

When sight is lost though the pupil is still bright, or even if it is dull, or if obstruction of the nerve has caused this ill, then, lest it be affected by yet other humours, quickly give pills of coccia or so-called pills of light to purify the brain. And then apply cups to the shoulders and caustic beneath the ear: and let fowl and thyme be well chewed. Try powdered hellebore and pyrethrum in the nostrils: apply a bonnet to the head to sweat the skin well in a steam-bath: or give draughts of guaiac, china root or sarsaparilla. Even the blind will have their sight restored by this liquor. Take pimpernel, celandine, fennel, vervain, germander, sage, celery and rue, knotgrass, the clove pink: and take an ounce of juice of each of these, and the same amount of flour, with added pepper, nutmeg and wood of aloes: and give three drachms at a time. And mix all this in a child's urine and add a sixth of the amount of malmsey, and place in a stoppered vessel, and instil one or two drops in the eye last thing at night. Excessive sleep is not good and roast food is best: and honey-water, and wine mixed with the herb eye-bright.

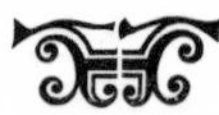

CHAPTER XIX

Remedies Indicated to Fortify the Eyes

Often the merest trifle offends the gentle eye, subject to every kind of ill, but it is invigorated by powerful herbs: fennel, celandine, rue, calendis, with pride of place to eye-bright or euphrasia. Prescribe liver and gall of goat, gall of partridge, crane, ashed viper's head and magpie, the brain of bat and swallow. Take the eyes of crab, cat, wolf, crow and magpie. Vision is sharpened when the ears are pierced: and the frequent sight of emerald and sapphire gives new strength to tired eyes, for they are rejoiced by blue and green: but to cure them, if red or sombre, instil the blood of turtle-dove or pigeon.

CHAPTER XX

Treatment of Inflammation of the Ear

When fever is linked with piercing pain in the ear, the danger is greater the more it is felt internally: and that the patient should not be soon afflicted by the frenzy, first give a suppository or an enema, and open the median vein and the cephalic too repeatedly, if the patient's strength allows. Gently purge the lower belly of the hot humours that afflict the brain: cup the shoulders and back and set on fire to extract excess heat from the site. First put warm oxyrhodium in the ear: and if the inflammation is severe, secure sound sleep with a decoction of rose and poppy: and, if you wish to relieve the pain, take a bag of mallow cooked with milk and apply when hot to the region of the painful ear. And if this does not relieve the pain and suppuration is desired, make a poultice of flax and flour of fenugreek with water and oil of goose and fowl. Cleanse the sore place with hydromel, or honey mixed with a bitch's milk, or syrup of wormwood and dried roses. Myrrh and Sabaean incense will regenerate the flesh. Let the diet be wholly liquid, the drink watered wine.

CHAPTER XXI

Treatment of Flatus and Obstruction of the Ear

Sometimes the phlegm or flatus gives rise to earache, and either may render deaf. Therefore, when the ear is oppressed by tinnitus or heaviness, purge with pills of hyeris or the imperial Indian pill known as agaric, and then give juice of garlic, leek and onion all together: and infuse rue and bitter almond in castor-oil and, when hot, instil two or three comforting drops within the ear. Take wine or aqua vitae, a touch of colocynth, euphorbia, castoreum, and introduce by tube their vapour in the ear, and use marjoram and hellebore as snuffs. And if this does not suffice, an infusion of lignum vitae may be helpful, or Vigo plaster made with mercury applied to neck and shoulders. Put honey in the drink to give a vinous odour: spice white bread with aniseed: let meat be roasted, such as pigeon, pheasant, partridge, done with skill: and fat sheep which nourishes so many.

CHAPTER XXII

Treatment of the Mumps

When it first develops, it is unwise to try to suppress the mumps, but if pain presses apply what is bland and gentle to the swollen part: the whey of butter is helpful, or oil pressed from sweet almonds, or camomile together with white lilies, or lanolin if you wish. Prescribe a poultice of wheat-flour, flax seeds with hydromel, barley and fenugreek: or in hydromel infuse mallow, camomile, marshmallow. And the fat of pig and calf helps to soften and lead to suppuration, as does that of fowl or goose, though its value is less certain if too hot: or use old oil or fat. And these remedies best relieve when the swelling is at its height and nature's forces focus the pestiferous humour here: and this can be drawn thither with powder of cantharides, and pigeon's dung, infused root of dittany mixed and fermented with marshmallow and delicate laurel oil. But if this fails to yield pus or resolve the humour, cauterize the lower part of the painful swelling: but first open a vein if the humour swells and relax the bowel with an effective remedy.

BOOK SEVEN

CHAPTER I

Treatment of Disorders of the Nose

If a polyp obstructs the nostrils and blunts the sense of smell, and if neither aqua fortis nor mercurial powder nor vitriol serves to remove it, it must be cut out with the knife: but complete removal is not assured if an ulcer develops, for this may become malignant. But touch the residue with lead ointment, nightshade, rose-water: and if the nasal stench is due to venereal disease, remedy with guaiac powder, hesperidium and honey. A stinking ulcer at the entrance to the nostrils causes ozaena and is due to venereal disease, cured as follows. If the humour is frankly devouring, growing apace and putrescent, take the sharp, sweet, austere juices of the pomegranate, mixed together, and rub into the affected part frequently: but if the flesh be soft and an ulcer forming, powdered dried roses should be used. And it is quite helpful for chronic coryza to make pastilles of myrrh, varnish and benzoin, mastic, incense, roses or soft resin containing turpentine, so that the nostrils may exhale the vapour from the live coals above. However, before touching this affection locally, it may be necessary to purge the body of its impure humours: and when it is the brain that is occupied by the cause of the disorder, this must be cleansed by frequent draughts and pills to secure that the peccant bile or corrupt humour is downwardly dispatched.

CHAPTER II

Treatment of Bleeding from the Nose

Whether bleeding from the nose is habitual, or comes in episodes, it may be that bleeding from periods or piles has ceased and that the epistaxis is protective: but arrest the flow of blood, if it is a symptom, by opening a vein in the elbow on the side that is bleeding, and the cephalic vein as well if the strength allows. Attach cups to shoulders and buttocks: apply a poultice to the forehead made up of many astringents, such as the Armenian bole, clay and volatile white flour, with juice of roses and sticky white of egg. The plaster used for hernia is a good defence or red desiccant or spider's web. Let the patient gradually smell the stink of ass's dung: nettles, leeks and camphor draw fluid from the nose: it is useful to apply oxycrat to liver and pudenda, and worth keeping this in the mouth. Best not to lie on a featherbed but on firm straw, nor prone, which allows blood exit from the nose, but supine: and apply ligatures to the limbs with frequent downward massage. Syrup of myrtle, rose and pomegranate, and oxycrat in julep, are good to drink: also conserve of comfrey and roses can be used, with added powder of red coral, sugar and quince juice. Broths to thicken thin blood are cooked with lettuce and with purslane: wine is forbidden, but water, pure or mixed with pink julep, makes a drink not unsuited to this disorder.

CHAPTER III
Treatment of Toothache

Because of their nerves, the teeth are affected by the most frightful pain, which can be abolished only by opening a vein and gentle purging, two measures to be used first against this ill. Let root of bitter capers be boiled in vinegar with oak-galls: or else use acrid colocynth or lousewort with hot pyrethrum or cold henbane to foment the tooth: for cold things blunt the nerve while caustics burn it. Hence, both heat and excessive cold abolish feeling: therefore, place oil of vitriol, laterum, thyme or seeds of opium on the carious tooth. Extract of china root rapidly inhibits the pain, or oil of amber: but to stop discharge, brace the temples with a poultice of Armenian earth and white of egg, or the red plaster used to desiccate. If the tooth is eroded or loose, or pain recurs often, it is better to extract it with an iron instrument.

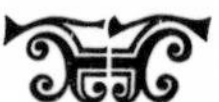

CHAPTER IV

Treatment of Perverted Taste, Stammering and Palsy of the Tongue

If depravity of taste impairs and embitters the tongue's response to savours, purge away the bile: and if the humours are tainted with salt or acid, excite a flux of phlegm or black fluid from the bowel. If, in stammering, the flow from the bowel is inadequate, arouse the downward flow of phlegm with diaphanicum or other familiar agents. To induce sweating of the entire body, infuse guaiac wood or sarsaparilla: if there is plethora, open the median vein, and then the vein that stores the moisture of the tongue. A like treatment is to be used for paralysis of the tongue: and if the cause of fluxion is in the head, dry with powdered amber, roses, sandalwood, varnish, incense, mace, styrax, musk and Indian nard, lemon-rind, schoenanthum, benzoin: sprinkle these on white gauze, place in a cap and apply this to the head. Apply the cautery to the neck, or ointment of the fox or castoreum oil: and have the patient chew French lavender, with added galingale, sage and rosemary, made up to the measure required by the catarrh.

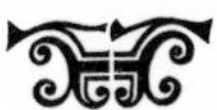

CHAPTER V

Treatment of Inflammation of the Tonsils and of the Uvula

Sometimes the tonsil becomes inflamed: and, lest it spread, be quick to bleed, first at the elbow and then the vein that drains the tongue. Apply cups to the neck and beneath the chin, after frequent scarification of the skin: wash out the mouth and throat with oxycrat or plantain water: rose-water too is useful, or water mixed with oak-gall and alum, juice of mulberry or of pomegranate seeds. Use enemas often and judge from the stools whether to purge the bile. The uvula is to be treated likewise: and, if unhealed, should not be cut with an instrument unless it dangles like a thin tail: for its division diminishes the voice, and loss of vital force spreads to all parts.

CHAPTER VI

Treatment of the Quinsy

When a swelling develops in the throat and gives rise to a quinsy, prescribe an enema and then open a vein such as the median or one beneath the tongue: and gargle in the manner we have described above, or with water infused with raisins, pomegranate, roses, cypress nuts. If there is pain, add milk of ass or cow or goat, or a little fenugreek. If the patient is choking, draw the swelling outwards with cupping-glasses applied to neck and chin, or suck it out with wool soaked in warm oil of lily or camomile: or apply a poultice of swallows' nests: or smear powder of millipedes and honey on the neck. If the mouth can be opened, let a crust of bread be swallowed: or a sponge fixed to a thread passed down the throat to where the swelling is will rupture it, and let the pus escape through the mouth with the aid of cough and tongue, the patient prone with head downwardly inclined. Fasting is helpful in this disease: but if the condition does not subside, sustain with hydromel or water, broths expressed from meat, and thin jellies.

CHAPTER VII

Remedies Against Diseases of the Chest

Those remedies that may be used for diseases of the chest include the following: sweet plums, the liquid cream from swollen barley, milk of sweet almonds, jujube with myxis, pine kernels, tragacanth, liquorice, gum-arabic, the white seeds of the silk-cotton tree, gentle mallow, the filbert, pistachio and honey, the juice of sugarcane: all can alleviate or prevent the fury of the bile. To cleanse, attenuate and clear the chest of phlegm, use raisins, figs, hyssop and maidenhair, safflower seed, white horehound, the small fern, potent gentian root, onion, garlic, leek, germander useful for the heart, ginger, origanum and calamint, thyme, savory, iris root, bitter dracunulus, arum, squill, saffron: all these herbs are usually effective. Use with myrrh and comfrey, coltsfoot, mint, scabious and pimpernel which absorbs pus and arrests its flow. The lung of fox and terebinth dry up the ulcers of the lung and inhibit dire spread of the consumption.

CHAPTER VIII

Treatment of Cough

The lung strives by coughing to empty what is hidden in its cavities. If little or nothing is spat out, the cough is dry: the humour is viscid or thin, fuelled by fires of fever, drying the windpipe. If, then, the humour is viscid, give infused hyssop or cleansing oxymel: if thin, thicken with syrup of rose and violet and poppy, and penidium, and tablets of tragacanth. If the windpipe is sore, relieve with milk or oil of sweet almonds, or the white liquor expressed from barley, liquorice, seeds of silcotton or mallow, infused with sugar-water. And add plum or sweet jujube. But if excess of humour burns the throat, then give horehound, calamint, iris or squill as linctus, hyssop or maidenhair.

CHAPTER IX

Treatment of Asthma

The broth of an old cock with leek relieves asthma: and senna with figs, liquorice, coltsfoot, origanum, thyme and added diacatharmus:

or hyeris or the invigorating agaric. And give syrups to rid the chest of phlegm: horehound, hyssop, thyme and maidenhair, and a little sulphur if the humour is sticky, also expelled in the sweat by lignum vitae. But that the phlegm should not form again, keep the patient in a soft bed, breathing warm air in a lofty room, or travelling in the country in an open carriage or in a tall ship on the seas: and let eating and drinking be restrained. However, do not proscribe what delights the palate: in fact, roast partridges and pigeon, fowl and turkey, all birds and four-footed beasts grateful to the stomach: and refined flour, twice-cooked, spiced with salt, coriander and fennel: and let but little wine be drunk, and that old, or potent mead which smells of wine. Usefully apply the cautery to the nape and the middle of the chest, and cupping-glases to both breasts and the loins towards the spine.

CHAPTER X

Treatment of Suffocating Catarrh

If the catarrh rapidly affects the throat and suffocates, open a vein without delay for delay is usually dangerous: and then give a strong enema to reduce the fierceness of the humour. And, to relieve the breathing, for drink give aqua vitae with sugar, honeyed squill, betony water, thyme, hyssop and cassia infusion. Cup the neck with a small flame. If this is not effective, purge as in asthma: and, whatever be the cause, the symptoms may be so severe as to bring us to our last brief hours.

CHAPTER XI

Treatment of Peripneumonia

In peripneumonia, to relieve the inflammation of the lung, first give a suppository to bring out the faeces: open a vein, lest the humour flow anew, and to open the narrowed channels that conduct the air: and do not hesitate to bleed again if breathing is hampered or fever is burdensome, but assay three or four times unless faintness supervenes. Then purge with cassia, lenitive or manna, senna and prunes, it the bowel is costive. For expectorants, give jujube, syrup of violets: or effect this with coltsfoot, liquorice, hyssop, maidenhair. Prescribe a tisane or sugared water or infusion of raisins with liquorice added: and a good diet consists of eggs and broth or jelly made from veal and capon. A liniment of oil of sweet almonds or of camomile relieves pain in the chest, as does a poultice of marshmallow, butter, flax, flour and fenugreek.

CHAPTER XII

Treatment of Empyema

After peripneumonia, abscess, pain in the side or quinsy and remission of previous pain, if there is heaviness and rigor it is followed by suppuration. And, lest delay lead to spreading damage in the chest and lay the basis for consumption, give that which enables sputum to be expelled by cough. And to soften hardness, give the following: violet and sebesten, the herb called coltsfoot, jujube, silk-cotton seed, penidia, the sweet root of liquorice. The pus is best drawn out by hyssop, maidenhair and oxymel, calamint and horehound, whose juices are made into a linctus with sugar. To expel the sputum, drink tisanes, oxymel, hydromel mixed with thyme: the diet should be as stated formerly. Senna itself is less acceptable, unless infused with plums, myxis, violets or sweet raisins, or with fat broth. Manna is innocuous and cassis mixed with terebinth softens and overcomes all humours, digests and purges out the pus. If still the heaviness does not yield, foment externally with oil and water, or water with gentle herbs like flowers of mallow, marshmallow, camomile all infused together: or try a poultice of figs, mallow, marshmallow, leek and dung of pigeons, with grease of pig, calf and goose, all cooked slowly with gum tragacanth. Hippocrates opened the side with an iron instrument or burned with fire, but you would do better to use the cautery. If the disease should linger on, but without fever, the milk of goat or ass may prove effective.

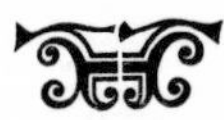

CHAPTER XIII

Cure of Phthisis, or Consumption

This consumption is called phthisis in Greek, and is associated with wasting and slow fever and severe ulceration of the lung: a disorder not to be overcome, for the cough required to cleanse the ulcer also lacerates the lung, which never eases moving and is barely susceptible to medication. The cause of the disorder is often in the head: therefore the way to act is to purge and support the brain, as already stated in connection with catarrh. Make sweet emulsions to be sipped with syrup of horehound, violet and maidenhair and whatever is needed to shift the sputum. Raisins are good to eat, and pine kernels, pistachio, fig, dates, the white juice of almonds preserved in sugar, and cream of barley. Express the juice of veal and use the jellied juices of various meats, the distillate of slow-footed turtles and of cray-fish, with a brace of partridges or chickens, a capon, conserve of borage mixed with that of roses, irises and violets, with powder of herb margaret, Armenian bole, tragacanth and coral. Woman's milk has pride of place, sucked from the breast as does a child: ass's milk has value here, goat's milk takes third place and cow's comes last: all nourish rapidly, cleanse out the pus, alleviate the fierce humour and close the lesion. And the powdered lung of fox should be taken in coddled eggs: and tisanes to drink with added plantain water or pink sugar-water, of a few drops of thin wine with much water added infused with pimpernel. Let baths be taken, but it is proper to eat first lest the patient faint while in the water. If the bowel be sluggish, give an enema with emollient herbs, milk, whey and salt: or give broth of an old cock, or manna by the mouth, or black cassia. Sleeplessness and care, grief and fear, anger, labour, the harmful rays of the sun, and cold: all these are noxious: but moderate warmth is useful and dry air, complete rest and sleep at night, and airs sung by sweetly modulated voices.

CHAPTER XIV
Treatment of Pleurisy

True pleurisy is of rapid onset and not without risk of death if the work is not carried out quickly. Therefore, for the pain in the side and difficulty in breathing and the acute fever, open an elbow vein, and do so often if the first or second bleeding has no effect. And if the bowel be sluggish, arouse it with suppository or enema: and prescribe by mouth gentlest cassia and manna or whatever is expectorant: the juice or root of liquorice, syrup of jujube, coltsfoot, ground ivy which is the famed cat's-foot, syrup of poppy, purple violet flowers and maidenhair, whey newly expressed from butter to be sipped: all gradually pervade the pathways of the lung. The white cream of sweet almond, sugared cream of barley and broth and jelly of capon, fowl and veal all reinvigorate and open the paths within the chest. Or tisanes of sugar-water may be drunk, and if the bladder is full of milk it relieves the pain: give every kind of fat and foment with poultices of camomile and marshmallow. If these do not suffice, divert the course of the humour elsewhere with lenitive and senna: or give whatever remedies may purge, like prunes. Massage the legs and bind the arms: and, if the periods or haemorrhoids are suppressed, open the saphenous vein or one that stands out knotty behind the knee: but first of all, open the arm veins on the side nearest the disease. If the false pleurisy is induced by flatus, apply to that side a bag filled with origanum, calamint and thyme: or foment the side with wool soaked in oil of laurel, terebinth or pennyroyal. And if the bitter humour is stagnant, rouse with an enema and give pills or other proper purges by the mouth. Apply cupping-glasses to the part: and if the pain presses, and excess of blood is evident, remove a part by section of a vein.

CHAPTER XV

Remedies for the Heart, or Cardiacs

Every kind of ill and every kind of poison, and the plague, attack the heart, damage and may destroy it unless it be defended with the powerful weapons known as cardiacs. Powdered Indian ivory, horn of unicorn and bezoar of repute: red Lemnian earth and Armenian bole, green emerald, pearl, sparkling sapphire and the stone called hyacinth, camphor, coral, that Venetian juice for which all thirst, and silver and metallic gold: all these work well. Water restrains the unbridled rages of the heart, and cuckoo's bread which is the wood sorrel we call oxytriphillum, borage, bugloss, flowers of violet and rose, juice of limes or yellow lemons and pomegranate: all of golden reputation, redolent with fragrance. And a juice that is particularly useful is that expressed from quince, and juice and seeds of sorrel that counter the lethal bite of scorpion. And for those cold ills that follow the hot humours, use nard of blessed fragrance and sharp costus, amomum, varicoloured wood of aloes, dappled cinnamon, saffron and the clove-pink beloved of the gods, lemon-rind, amber and musk that pleases more than any other odour, the seed weavers use for their red dye, tormentil short in leaf but great in power, blessed cardoon and not unwelcome balm, succusa and like leaves arising from the elm, what was called turnix and now bistort or snakeweed, and the dittany that grows on Mount Ida: and seeds of zedoary, galingale, angelica, germander, scabious: and these are usually swallowed or else applied to the body and pierce and destroy the plague.

CHAPTER XVI

Treatment of Palpitations of the Heart

When a delicate heart trembles and quavers terrifyingly, in what the Greeks called *palmon,* there is some risk of death unless you quickly help. Therefore determine whether excess of blood may cause this ill, or that the blood is too hot, or whether bile is the cause or else a heavy drowsy vapour, or if it is a swelling introduced into the heart, perhaps born of putrescent matter or of thick air that fills and distends: or whether the membrane that clothes and invests the heart is everywhere inundated with fluid so that the heart palpitates excessively, or that the blood is overheated – for this bleed profusely, but less so if there is some other cause. In all other cases, however, you must open the vein at the outset: nor omit to purge, to bind the limbs or cup, or open the veins at the ankle or behind the knee to withdraw the humour which is, or may be, noxious. Give manna and rhubarb if the cause is heat, and whey with senna if it is the black humour. If there is excess of phlegm or wind, a dilute infusion of white agaric in wine quickly reinvigorates. Musk and amber, Galen's powder and hippocras, quickly warm and arouse the forces oppressed and overcome by cold. If due to devouring fire, water of wood-sorrel is indicated, with syrup of lemons or apples: also alchermes and herb margaret, amber and precious stones. The wood of aloes is useful for destructive causes:

and of course mithridatum and theriac are cardiacs that can be used for both beverage and fomentation, or as an opiate bolus. Let the atmosphere be free, serene and pleasantly fragrant, the mind untroubled and sleep moderate, the bowels opened naturally or by art, and the meals restrained. However, to restore the forces give broths, distillates and jellies: and the spirits soar with mountain or forest birds as victuals, and such fowl as partridge, cock or turkey. If heat is intense, try the divine drink: otherwise, water mixed with wine will do no harm.

CHAPTER XVII
Treatment of Syncope

To overcome syncope, and to recall the spirit from the darkness where it has wandered, fill the mouth with wine, let the nose sense vinegar, and for food give broths, distillates and jellies, which are readily absorbed. And, to restore the exhausted spirits and expel the dire poisons and digest the humours, give imperial drink or theriac water or extract of bark of cinnamon. If the face and pulse give grounds for hope, eliminate the cause of this abrupt collapse. If it is excess of blood, fever or oppressed breathing, and if the strength allows, open a vein. If there is excessive bile or a sour humour, let a mild enema be given: or give manna, senna or rhubarb as cardiacs: if phlegm is a burden, add those agents we have described to dislodge the phlegm. If the stomach is sensitive, a savage air from different parts strikes the heart: or severe pain, violent exertion or immoderate internal flux, sleeplessness, grief, anxiety or pestiferous air: all these may cause collapse and are to be combatted by their contraries. Foment the head with water of balm or sorrel, sweet basil, the triple sandalwood and musk and camphor, and Panchaian amber added for its odour. Or take conserve of roses, violets, balm and water-lily: and unequalled theriac and mithridatum, amber and precious stones: or make a poultice with rosewater or vinegar to apply to the region of the heart: give water of sorrel, devil's-bit or scabious to drink, together with powdered bezoar, sweet lime syrup and prepared alchermes: and precious stones and herb margaret.

CHAPTER XVIII

Treatment of Haemoptysis or Spitting Blood

If there is a flow of foamy red blood from lung or chest, open a vein lest phthisis follow: nor should one gasp, but breathe gently, keep silent, feast little and drink syrup of barberry, rose, myrrh or red currant, or the purple juice of pomegranate seeds. If the prime cause of this disorder is downward flow of catarrh, cleanse the brain with pills and potions, and then apply the skull-cap as described above. Apply cold to the liver, it will withdraw poison from afar: and rub the limbs and bind them firmly. Coral, haematite, Lemnian earth, mummy, stag's horn, gleaming pearl, and myrrh, incense, spodium, amber, tragacanth, dragon's blood and Armenian bole and the three sandalwoods: all serve to close the gaping vessels and can be prepared in various ways: made into a powder to be mixed with milk or yolk of egg, or compressed into a tablet. The corn-poppy freezes and condenses a fierce humour and should be given when a vessel has been eroded.

BOOK EIGHT

CHAPTER I

Remedies Pleasing to the Stomach, Known as Stomachics

If heat affect the stomach and lead to vomiting and loss of appetite, give cherry, oxyacanth, red currant and pomegranate, medlar, serviceberry, quince and those remedies that flourish under the sun: myrrh and fresh olives, citinus, flower of wild pomegranate, sorrel and red rose, coriander seed, coral, ivory hardened in fire, licium, cistus and hypocystis and acacia: all those that suppress vomiting and excessive menstrual flow. If the stomach wall is infiltrated with a cold humour, let it be warmed and thinned and its strength restored with both kinds of mint, wormwood, sage, spikenard, saffron, mastic, wood of Indian aloes. Give fuscum, mace and nutmeg, galanga, bark of cinnamon, cloe and hot ginger and amber of outstanding fragrance, myrobalan and those tears the poplar sheds into the river Erydanum that harden under water.

CHAPTER II

Treatment of a Weak Stomach

If the stomach languishes because of fiery heat, forbid the drinking of cold beverages and give boiled water only or with bread immersed, or add bland syrup of barberry, pomegranate or rosewater. Prepare broths with lettuce, sorrel, capon, mutton, veal and young pigeons: also roast and boiled flesh, for excess of fluid weakens the stomach, so do not give these broths too often. Add the seeds of pomegranate to the food and give medlar, pear and quince after meals: if there is excess bile, give manna and rhubarb. Let the meals be small, for the stomach impaired by disease has little heat and so requires but little food, but oft repeated, so that the limbs may gradually regain their vigour. If the stomach is infirm and cold, it is harmful to drink water unless mixed with cinnamon and sugar: and redolent old wine is helpful and, with absinth added, cleanses, invigorates and restores lost appetite. Salt bread is good, and roast pigeon, turtle-dove, pheasant, lark, partridge, thrush, turkey and other well-known birds. If phlegm harms the stomach, purge with pills of bitter aloes: aromatic confection of roses, taken before meals, strengthens. Foment with fragrant calamus, wormwood, mint, marjoram, roses and coarse wine, and rub in afterwards with oil of roses, mastic, spikenard, nutmeg and mint, using a goose-feather gently applied to the belly or the skin of hare or rapacious vultures or the fleece of sheep. Sleep will usually digest the crude humours, tame excessive heat and is therefore good. Anxiety and anger are to be avoided.

CHAPTER III

Treatment of Cholera

Cholera, so-called, is a sharp and savage disorder: therefore it is surely best not to restrain this rage or to suppress the bilious humour that causes this fierce ill. But if excessive vomiting becomes exhausting it should be checked with pomegranate juice or syrup of red currant, myrrh or roses. Foment the stomach with powdered sandalwood, red roses or coral, with a little camphor in rosewater and added vinegar. Rub in oil of myrrh, reinforced with mastic, and powder of white ivory: the application of a single tablet will suppress the vomiting. But lest this ill, unchecked, furiously return, harry the bile downward in the belly, provided only that excessive flux and pain do not oppress and destroy vitality. Give an enema of water boiled with roses, houseleek, plantain, mallow, lettuce. Apply wine to the nostrils and give water mixed with wine to drink to numb and occlude the flow of humour. Bind the hands and feet and apply a large cupping-glass to the belly for a long time. If the limbs become cold and convulsed, rub with a hot towel: if there is vomiting or flux, suppress either by copious bleeding, which alleviates severe pain and dislodges bile and fiery heat. However, if this violent disorder does not yield, give a pill of dog's-tongue or philonium as an antidote to ensure sound sleep: if sleep comes, it checks the bile and restrains all fluxions except the sweat.

CHAPTER IV

Remedies Peculiar to the Liver, or Hepatics

Purslane relieves pains in head and stomach, and lettuce checks the fierce and bitter bile that seizes on the liver: but the liver gains more support from endive, all kinds of sorrel, plantain, the lichen known as liverwort, dog's-tooth grass, and seeds or roots of whatever is cold. Ivory, spodium, roses, sandalwood and coral refresh the inflamed liver: but if the distress is due to inclement cold humour, take root of asparagus and parsley, good for the menses, fennel, seeds of whatever is heating like hop and maidenhair, wormwood, agrimony that dispels slow fever, and gout-relieving ivy and cassutha, germander, hog's fennel, fumitory that clarifies the humours and the blood, the fragrant rush called calamus, and galingale: and raisins usually relieve the liver, whether it be hot or cold.

CHAPTER V

Treatment of Obstruction of the Liver

The thick humour that obstructs the liver is to be expelled downwards through the anus by injection of an enema: and drink, diluted with water, dog's-tooth grass, asparagus, butcher's broom, horehound, syrup of the roots of both endive and chicory, and maidenhair and oxymel. And cook together securidaca, agrimony leaves, senna and fennel seed and fern and wild celery: and infuse in this white agaric and two drachms of the rhubarb that grows wild at large: and thus dislodge and destroy the sluggish juices and expel them from the liver into the bowel. Or give pills of hyeris, made into a warm drink with diacatharmus water, horehound, mint, wild celery or parsley, and the result will be a well-chosen way of life, more delicate than overfull, for what is subtle gathers, resolves and digests the humours. And thereto let roast mountain birds be often taken, but not too many broths, and eat a little well-cooked bread. Drink but little wine or water, and take confection of red roses before meals, made with many aromatics, or dialacca or diacuruma will do instead. If the cause of the disorder is sticky phlegm, opening a vein is harmful: but this is not the case if there is bile or excess of humour.

CHAPTER VI

Treatment of Inflammation of the Liver

When the liver is aroused and swollen by inflammation, evacuate the bowel with a mild enema: and bleed freely, right away, from the right elbow, and if this does not succeed the first or second time, a third may relieve the pain.

Meanwhile, it is right to take purges for the noxious humours so as to withdraw the bitter bile: rhubarb is one, but I rate cassia highest, and manna and chicory mixed with hepatica water. But if there is not so much heat, or less abundant humour, diaprune or so-called lenitive is fit to blunt its fierceness. And then foment with rosewater, plantain, nightshade, endive and wormwood: with these waters you can mix powder of the three sandalwoods and spikenard and schoenantum, with vinegar a useful adjunct. Then make a liniment with oil that is not rancid or, if it is, purify with rosewater: and oxyrhodium is effective here, with oil of quince, wormwood, myrrh and rose: and, if you wish, add water of nightshade and houseleek and powder of dried roses. Give broths of flesh of veal, kid or turkey, using the entrails, and fresh raisins, dock and lettuce: and, for drink, give liquorice water with dog's-tooth grass, syrups of violet, myrrh, sorrel, lime and pomegranate, for these are usually grateful to the palates of the sick and extinguish the fire within.

CHAPTER VII

Treatment of Abscess of the Liver

Liver abscess is a swelling due to inflammation almost incapable of remedy: nevertheless, if there be a mode of cure, it is this. First inject an enema to restrain and dispel the vapours and the faeces gathered in the bowel: then bleed. Apply a poultice to the liver containing shepherd's purse and the side-shoots of vines and many roses, myrrh, evergreen, lettuce, gourds and heat-giving wormwood with plantain: and make a liniment of their oils and juices and apply hot as liniment and poultice. If you would purge, do not use strong remedies: black cassia expels the humours gently, and lenitive, Calabrian manna and whey, and add to these rhubarb but not the senna and, before every meal, that laudable cream of barley which cleanses and purges. Rose-sugar and dog's-tooth make useful tisanes that help to divert pus from the liver to the loins if a hump-back is involved, and in closing a devouring ulcer. And this can be done also with root of hundred-headed dog's-tooth, wild celery and fennel: but to these must be added agrimony and chicory, plantain, liverwort, sorrel, roses, the four seeds commonly known as smaller, and the larger too.

CHAPTER VIII

Treatment of Cirrhosis of the Liver

Cure cannot be guaranteed when the liver is the site of cirrhotic swelling: but as long as sensitivity and pain persist, the hope of recovery is not altogether vain. Therefore, if there is an accumulation of dense obstructing juices, open the pathways with wild celery, butcher's broom and fennel: infuse together senna and juice of white roses and diacatharmus may be added, or diaphenicum, which rapidly expel from the bowel what otherwise would linger stubbornly. If there is fever and the veins are distended, open them, but not if the distension is by wind instead of blood: if winds there are, they rapidly subside when the vessel is opened, therefore refrain from letting excess of blood and coapt the gaping wound in the vein. But, to soften this hard scirrhus, take marrow of deer and calf and goose's fat: and if you wish also to strengthen the cirrhotic liver, add to these the cerate composed of the three sandalwoods, nard, wormwood, rose and cold-dispelling myrtle: and a little vinegar is not amiss to secure more penetration, or wine if the scirrhus is caused by a tenacious humour. And the best support is that of a soft and moist regime, secured by flesh of kid, calf and fowl: and give liquorice to drink.

CHAPTER IX

Treatment of Debility of the Liver

If the liver is langourous and its powers waver, strengthen by fomentation with roses, the fragrant reed calamus and wormwood: and make a liniment with oil of mastic, rose and myrtle: or, instead of these, use cerate containing the three sandalwoods. With ten times as much sugar, make tablets from powdered ivory, spodium, spikenard, myrrh, saffron, bark of cinnamon, coral and pearl, horn of stag and unicorn, and red roses together with the three sandalwoods and grains of musk. But you must add to this powder of wolf's liver, right to reinvigorate the liver. If heat is excessive, prepare an aposema of chicory, endive and sorrel, dog's-tooth, cold seed-corn and soft raisins. If a purge is wanted, add tamarind and rhubarb. If the disorder is cold, do the same with wormwood and germander and root of fern, wild celery or parsley, and purge with rhubarb and bright yellow terebinth. Roast partridge is good, and pigeon, but snails are famous: do without wine if feverish: it is better to drink pink sugar-water or barberry infusion or pomegranate juice. If it is a cold cause, infused agrimonary is helpful, and wine need not be forbidden, provided it is well diluted with water.

CHAPTER X

Remedies for the Spleen, or Splenics

Bugloss and sweet-smelling violet comfort the spleen, as do hop, hart's-tongue, dodder, bark and leaves of tamarisk, dock, fruit of caper and its root and bark, germander, squill, galingale, root of wild celery and red radish and fern infused in oxymel, and polypody root to dislodge the black juices: and hog's fennel, willow, agrimony, iris, the lesser centaury, cyclamen, lamb's lettuce, rue and stinging nettle, mustard which attracts the thick humour from afar and relieves all kinds of pains: soapwort and the drops commonly called lac, gum ammoniac together with bdellium, of which take little if not macerated in vinegar: and use all these to make a plaster for the soft spleen with wax and oil of caper or of rue. And, that a smile may move the spleen, make tablets with Galen's powder or precious stones with herb margaret.

CHAPTER XI

Treatment of Splenetics, That is, Those Whose Spleen is Tense and Hard

If the spleen is tense and hard and burdened, first inject an enema, next purge repeatedly with lenitive or hamech, and added diaprune: and often senna, but uncooked as we have said before about the spleen: and such as bugloss, hop, hart's-tongue, bark of caper, and add fennel and wild celery, which dispel the winds that vex and swell the spleen. If they are distended and bleeding is indicated, make a wide opening in the veins: first cut the basilic and later the cephalic: venesection is indicated for the spleen, but if you are fearful apply leeches, attach cupping-glasses and often boldly scarify to draw off the black blood. Rub over the spleen with goose-fat, calf-marrow and oil of rue, or else with ointment made of powdered scale-fern with frankincense and ammoniac, dissolved in vinegar: inunct the region where you feel the swelling. Make tablets of iron, scale-fern, coral, tamarisk, wood of cinnamon and powdered spikenard with sugar added: one drachm to be swallowed in the early morning, another in the evening: and drink ash mixed with wine and water in a vessel which, infused, lightens the spirits and removes care and provides sleep: but chalybeate water is more useful, more allegrative. For morning eating, give birds roasted or boiled with parsley, hyssop, thyme and other warming herbs: for, if the spleen be not altogether scirrhous, it requires a bland and tepid diet. The spleen of ass, fowl or horse: the body of a bat with head removed: these are suitable for the black humour of the spleen.

CHAPTER XII

Treatment of Hypochondriac Melancholy

In hypochondriac disease, force the dark humour downwards with frequent enemas. Infuse mallow and marshmallow and other gentle herbs with seeds of dill and fennel and senna, and let this be taken with prunes often, or with fat broths. And hamech is helpful, and lenitive and black cassia from India: polypody and beet boiled with a cook: diaprune and whey: and take a drachm of bark of black hellebore, of hyeris and seed of colocynth, pills of fumitory, lapis lazuli. The humour is usefully alleviated by hop and lettuce, dog's-tooth and asparagus, scalefern and maidenhair and borage, bugloss, liquorice, mallow and purslane, plain hydromel or oxymel, syrup of jujube, fumitory or maidenhair and violet, and vinegar of famous flavour and most evil smell. Bleed often if the veins are swollen, the liver hot, the patient young, the menses absent: but only rarely if this is not the case. Fomentations to the hypochondriac regions give no small relief when they contain the odorous galingale and spikenard and aromatic calamus, thyme and dodder, origanum, calamint, camomile, melilot, seeds and root of sweet cyperus, all in more water than wine. And make a liniment from the oils of caper and violet, nard, wormwood and mild camomile: and warm bathing is helpful for the most furious anxiety if the skin be dry.

CHAPTER XIII

Treatment of Disorders of the Mesentery

When the mesentery is affected by many humours, and if the cause of the disorder is not apparent to you elsewhere, then place your hand there: and if you feel it hard, apply all your remedies at that site. If there is a considerable slow fever, first inject an enema, open a vein, then delay to see if the remedy is effective in drawing out the humours down below, and this should be repeated quite often with senna. If the obstruction is of long standing and does not yield, add what will thin the thick matter and hasten it from the bowel, like diacatharmus, benedict, hyeris and diaphenicon: but, with any remedy, purge in relation to its force and the patient's temperament. And, for a fomentation, rose, mint, mallow, cyperus, prepared root of mallow, calamint and thyme are suitable.

CHAPTER XIV

Treatment of Jaundice

The jaundiced should not be allowed to work, or to be gnawed by care, but lie in a soft bed and sleep in a well-lighted room: he should sing, dance and jest and feast sumptuously and water his wine. Let him be neither hot nor cold and inhale soft air and let draughts be excluded: and if a better, warmer fluid circulates in the body than before, the bile will cease to form. And to evacuate this, first give an enema, and then open a vein if there is also fever and heat, or if the menses have ceased as often seen in girls or widows. Purge as required with lenitive and syrup of white roses: and if the gallbladder or liver are blocked and swollen, open the pathways with attenuating herbs such as wild celery, calamint and chicory, caper and radish, anchusa, germander, maidenhair, agrimony, hop, gentian that rapidly restores the menses, ivy and horsehound, fern, fennel, thyme, the roots of endive and of maidenhair, syrup of china root, the simple oxymel called squill of which prepare an apozeme. And if you desire discharge from the bowel, give diacatharmus or one or other hyeris to relieve, benedict, white agaric, or pills of hyeris or aloes, myrrh and saffron, or pills of light to be swallowed on the midnight. And when all that was obstructed is relaxed, follow with baths, which by themselves serve to overcome the jaundice when, at the crisis, the torrid bile, firmly adherent to the skin, deposits there its fury without fever. If the skin has newly taken up the poison, to ingest fat will vomit out the jaundice, and then drinking milk will blunt its forces. If a serpent's fang has caused this lesion, withdraw the bitter venom by means of cupping-glasses, or apply leeches to the blemish: or give grains of bezoar with water of cardoon. The golden oriole should be viewed during this disorder: and give saffron, fruit of winter-cherry, filings of Indian ivory and sulphur taken in coddled eggs. It is said that this poison is corrected by the skin: but let reason decide the cause of the disorder.

CHAPTER XV

Treatment of Cachexia, or Poor Physical Condition

Three kinds of wasting are listed: their names are atrophy, when the torpid body declines nourishment: and phthisis is another, when emaciation accompanies an ulcer of the lung: and the foul cachexia troubles when the liver functions badly. We employ one and the same mode of treatment for both phthisis and atrophy: but in treating cachexia, beware of a possible attack of dreaded hydrops, unamenable to cure. Therefore, lest the body accumulate new excrement, and if nature is ineffective, relax the bowel with a suppository or enema and give pills of hyeris and ruffi, and wild rhubarb infused in water, wormwood and endive. And if rhubarb fails to purge, follow with draughts of white roses with senna added. It is useful to take curcuma and lacca and tablets of those aromatics that invigorate the stomach and liver. Simple food is best and food juices and watered wine. Natural water containing sulphur, alum and nitre is good as baths and drinks, for it attenuates, digests and alleviates all things.

CHAPTER XVI

Treatment of Dropsy

Of the three dropsies, the white does the least damage: the tympanites is greater, and worst of all is the ascites. And those remedies that expel the waters generally fortify and cure by reopening whatever channels are occluded and by desiccating. Therefore purge with agaric and pale roses, diacatharmus and colocynth, and those famous pastilles known as alhandal: and pills of spurge-flax, sweet-pea, sabucus: and cyclamen, dwarf-elder, wild cucumber and iris. And agents kind to liver and stomach are galanga and spikenard, bark of cinnamon, with added pepper, ginger, fennel, seeds of aniseed. Set free the water of the kidneys with nettle, radish, butcher's broom and maidenhair, fennel root, wild celery and parsley, dried and made into a powder. Massage vigorously, curtail food and drink, expose to the heat of the sun's rays and to dry air at sea or on the coast: frequent a blazing fire, bury the body in sand or corn, bathe in hot springs of sulphur, nitre or salt that issue from the earth: and, if nature does not provide these, imitate with hyssop, calamint, French lavender, fennel and marjoram, roses, juniper berries, fragrant thyme and laurel: all infused in water to which sulphur is added. Do not drink as much as thirst impels: and if thirst torments, oxycrat or liquorice to chew will soothe. From time to time a little weak white wine may be drunk and helps the power of the kidneys to get rid of water. Biscuit is to be eaten and roast birds. However, if the hydrops is seen to have its origin in heat and excessive thirst is intolerable, let the food be somewhat moister, roasted and boiled. If it is a cold disorder, venesection is impermissible: but if it is or once was febrile, or when there have been no periods or haemorrhoids, do not hesitate to bleed from the great vein at the elbow or to repeat at the knee or ankle. If the fluid is pooled in the abdomen, apply an ointment of spurge-laurel: or apply a poultice, usefully combined with sulphur or vesicants or black pyrotics, to the middle of the belly and scarify this region. But if health is not so to be restored, try paracentesis, a procedure always dubious and to be done only in the most dangerous situations. Place on the belly the stone vomited by a water-snake, and drink the fluid removed from one whose belly is so distended. If the skin is everywhere swollen up with phlegm, quina or sarsaparilla may be drunk to good effect.

CHAPTER XVII

Treatment of Ileus, or Volvulus

If volvulus obstructs the passage of faeces by the bowel, first inject a bland enema into the anus, made of mild flowers of camomile and mallow, and the grease of tripes, liquefied by heat if hard, with much salt. And then enquire what the cause of the disease may be. If it is heat, and bile, dislodge with laxatives such as diaprune or by opening a vein. Give hyeris for thick phlegm and make a poultice for the belly with linseed, mallow, grease of goose and calf. Gentle baths with infused camomile and other herbs are useful. Vomiting is indicated, but the best is for the bowel to act, unless it be that deadly poison has been taken, when one should be made to vomit and take bezoar. If the intestine has descended into the scrotum to cause this ileus, reduce this by manual force and rub in warm oil: and then it is proper to tie up the part that the disorder may not recur and prove fatal.

CHAPTER XVIII

Treatment of Colic

The pain of windy colic is to be relieved by enemas containing mint and rue and thyme, seeds of fennel, rue, bishop-weed and cumin, diaphenicum, salt, honey of the plant mercury, and oil of laurel and of dill. And let the fluid drunk be vinous hydromel or obtained from bark of cinnamon: and that kind of nut made from ginger and pepper helps. Foment the stomach with sachets of origanum and calamint and make a liniment of oil of rue or nuts. Apply an ample cupping-glass to the belly: the flame within will dissipate all winds and the frightful pain they cause. And if the origin be congealed or viscous phlegm, then give an enema: and afterwards a purge of mint, wild celery and such warming herbs, and infuse in this agaric, a remedy that draws out every humour, diacatharmus and laxative benedict, or hyeris, excess of which is bitter and unpleasant but succeeds often in expelling resistant noxious humours by the bowel. Let the diet be restricted and meagre, the wine old and mixed with wormwood and heated to invigorate all the adjacent parts: malvoisie and hippocras are agreeable and have a good effect on head and liver. Do not be afraid to open a vein, especially if the humour is both cold and abundant, for it is the best way out of this torment: and fomentation too suppresses pain. Immerse the body in a warm bath in which marshmallow leaves, melilot, dill and seeds of flax and camomile have been boiled: and these will surely succeed in getting rid of the bile from the colon, where it causes savage pains, faintness, spasms, cold sweats and fevers, and frequent vomiting of green and yellow bile. And hunger is also involved as a cause of this. Bland remedies will help: cassia, manna, rhubarb and food and drink that moisten. If the pain becomes excruciating and does not yield to these, induce refreshing slumber rapidly with pills of hyeris, of which give one drachm, or two drachms of castoria grains or numbing opium.

CHAPTER XIX

Treatment of the Lienteric and the Coeliac Flux

In the coeliac and the lienteric flux, the humour that gnaws the stomach lining is to be eliminated by pills of ruffi or hyeris and tablets of red rhubarb with the three sandalwoods. Then fortify the languid part with juices of quince, red currant, myrtle and pomegranate, infused with mint, rose, wormwood, sugar and various syrups, to be taken before meals. Or, as our fathers counselled for the sick, make up tablets from spikenard, red roses, spodium and saffron and rhubarb, wood of aloes, berberis, musk, mastic, gum-arabic and tragacanth. Take wormwood, rose, mint and nard and moisten as a fomentation with schoenanthum and fragrant cyperus, and use oil of nard as liniment. And I recommend Peruvian balsam mixed with Galen's cerate to protect the sensitive belly until its strength returns, laid on with linen. The food should be easily cooked: of all birds, the lark roasted is most relieving. Mix water with wine for drink: and end the meal with cooked quince or pear.

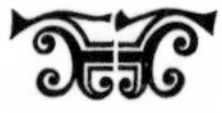

CHAPTER XX

Treatment of Diarrhoea

Sometimes potent nature is used to evacuate by the bowel, lightening the ballast of the loaded body: then, if all goes well in the following hours or days, the humour flows elsewhere. But if the flux persists, with pallor and weakened pulse, and appetite does not return and the anal flux continues, it must be rapidly suppressed to prevent languor of the stomach and the liver and parching dropsy. If there is fever and flow of bile, it helps to open a vein, but only bleed a little. Then let the three sandalwoods and rhubarb be swallowed: or infuse these with water of barberry, endive, plantain, drunk with liquor of pomegranate, myrtle or rose. Prepare an enema of roses and red dragon's blood, Armenian bole with scalded milk. And let the diet be light: roasts are most useful, and easily cooked victuals such as partridge, capon, fowl, thrush and tender pigeon. And the water drunk should contain iron, and one part of wine diluted with two parts of water.

CHAPTER XXI

Treatment of Dysentery

The cruel dysentery, accompanied by colic, is frequently excited by fierce bile and salty phlegm. It is appeased by syrup of violet with cassia: and use an enema of soft eggs with milk drawn from the distended udder of a cow. Give hulled barley and sweet almonds with sugar, soothing emollient broths of partridge and fat flesh of kid or capon, and the jelly that congeals from these and tender veal. But if these do not relieve completely, if the fever is constantly oppressive, if the body is stout and strong, if the menses cease and there is no other kind of flux, unhesitatingly cut the vein. Then purge with senna and rhubarb mixed with prunes, sebesten and raisins. The lenitive called synthesis is helpful, and sometimes diacatharmus can be added, but not too much, and less than usual of agaric unless the origin of the disease is salty phlegm and raw humours abound within the body. But do not confine the bowels before the noxious humour has been expelled, and unless the natural flux has caused undue weakness and excessive pain. Then the cold juices expressed from quince and barberry, rose and pomegranate, may be tried: and myrobalan, pear, sorb-apple, medlar, cornel-berry and rhubarb strongly pressed: or rhubarb mixed with the three sandalwoods, powdered ivory, horn of stag and unicorn: and one may burn sometimes. And make an enema of roses, willow, plantain, honeysuckle, houseleek, chilled seeds of psillium, lettuce and purslane, with red oak-galls: infuse all these and dissolve Armenian bole or Lemnian earth, alum or starch. If unremitting pain denies rest and sleep, give grains of soporific opium and philonium as antidote. Dry up the ulcer with vapours introduced through the anus:

of myrtle, red roses, cypress nuts, incense, wood of aloes, varnish, mastic, gum-arabic, terebinth obtained from trees. Let the meat be roast, and old red wine be drunk with barberry water, unless fever strongly contraindicates: and pink sugar-water is outstanding.

CHAPTER XXII

Treatment of Tenesmus

Who has tenesmus has rectal pain delayed until the end of defecation: and often, despite much effort, nothing is brought forth from the anus but a little mucus mixed with blood. It is often useful to give goat's milk: and purge with a bland remedy, but first soothe with an enema: and finally keep dry and warm until the excess phlegm is digested. For this take origanum, laurel, melilot, dill, rue and camomile to make a fomentation at the anus, and retain it there. Rub with liniment of warm oil of rue or laurel. The vapours of dry pitch, bitumen, pine nuts, and resin, well received, dry up the ulcer. If you require a cause for tenesmus and the dysentery, a thick phlegm is the best explanation I can offer.

CHAPTER XXIII

Treatment of Worms

Stomach worms prefer pleasant things as food: therefore do not drink milk or eat veal, eggs, fat broths, lest they crawl upwards and injure the stomach with their fierce bite, exciting spasm, syncope or death. Give by the anus honey prepared with milk, which dislodges the worm downward: and purge with rhubarb, hyeris, mint and purslane seed: again the worms give wormwood, pure or given as powder in water. The water drunk should be infused with sebesten and ivory and stag's horn added. Apply to the middle of the belly a plaster of pills of Ruffi prepared with honey. Mithdridatum with theriac is an antidote, and water of cardoon with whatever is bitter kills the cruel worms. And, as gluttony is their source, they are to be overcome by meagre diet and strenuous labour.

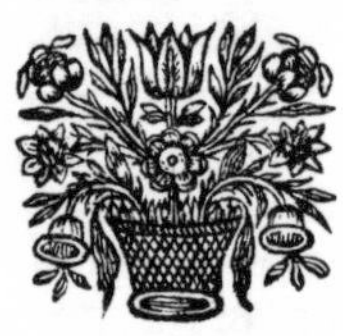

BOOK NINE

CHAPTER I

Nephritics, or Remedies Suited to the Kidneys

The kidneys suffer disorders caused variously: by infarction, inflammation, tumours, abscess, clots, ulcers, pus and stones. Jujube and plums relieve, and sweet almond, mallow root, strobilus, pistachio, fig, plums and cherries, tragacanth, black cassia, purple violet, liquorice, cream of barley, the red fruit of winter-cherry, all cold seeds both large and small, bramble and ginger, benign to stomach and kidney: and plantain, dog's-tooth, blackberry, sorrel, asparagus together with the herb called pellitory, lime juice, and the delicate maidenhair, water-lily flowers and, if the disorder is hot, seed of white poppy. If the passages are blocked with thick phlegm or stones or clot, open them with chickpea, pimpernel and herbs such as saxifrage, wild celery, marathrum, camomile land parsley and excellent hundred-headed cardoon, stinging-nettle, fragrant calamus, cyperus root, peony, ruscus, thousand-seeded sunflower, juniper and laurel berries and dazzling terebinth: and both of the star-thistles, rock samphire, cress, root and seed of wild carrot, black lovage and syon, radishes, broom, and the hazelwort that expels various humours, especially the phlegm.

CHAPTER II

Treatment of Weakness of the Kidneys

If the kidneys are weakened by distemper, whether simple or compound, occasioned by excessive running, long sitting on horseback, or by a fall or blow or by the circumstances previously described, pursue the contrary remedy. Cassia and rhubarb expel the heat from the kidneys: smear on cooling poplar ointment or the cerate Galen is said to have invented: and combat cold with clear turpentine, wormwood, roses and bland cyperus. Refrain from running and riding, avoid blows or falls on the back. It is bad to mix red wine with turbid water: let it be drunk clear. And if the veins, overfilled with blood, compress the emulgent vessels of the kidneys, first open the basilic vein and then the veins at the knee and ankle. Agents that hasten the passage of the urine weaken the kidneys: therefore divert the passage of the humours via the stools or skin so as not to deprive the kidneys of their strength. The jewstone invigorates, and the three yellow sandalwoods mixed with rhubarb, and tragacanth, and added ivory and rose and either form of coral: and rest is helpful, whatever be the cause. Prohibit any kind of work, and venery, and caressing baths which dilate the passages. The proper food is partridges, pigeons, fowls and doves, and the kidneys of other animals are very satisfactory. Ewe's milk is the first to try, and cream of barley mixed with starch. Medlars and service-berries help: and pears, quinces, cornelian cherry, whatever is astringent and reinforces the body's orifices: and barberry and chalybeate fluid mixed with water added to the best wine.

CHAPTER III

Treatment of Diabetes

When diabetes dries up the kidneys, there is oppressive panting thirst: for the water drunk but rarely is retained since the ingested fluid is quickly passed. Therefore, the fire that causes thirst must be extinguished, and the humour thickened: so administer whatever cures and cools and tempers. Sorrel is helpful here, and lettuce separately or cooked with fowl, veal or kid: and coddled eggs cooked in water. Milk known to be chalybeate is excellent, and cream of barley, and the juice of sweet almonds, and the cold seed of the corn-poppy. And make a nectar of those seeds called cold, or preserve of red currant and famed quince jelly. The juice of henbane, plantain and nightshade: the mucilage extracted from seeds that moistens the kidneys; and oil of myrtle or poplar, better with a little camphor: all these are of good effect. Make a poultice of barley, if you wish, and flour and oxyrhodium, and the juice of white poppy mixed with lettuce: or take Armenian bole and white of egg:

and if the liver is suffering from adjacent fire, foment with juices of endive, rose and plantain, and powdered sandalwood diluted with vinegar. But from the start open the veins daily, and give manna and tisane to drink, or black cassia, or tamarisk, white roses, rhubarb and senna. Syrups of myrtle, violet, rose, wild barberry and pomegranate are often grateful: and so is the water in which a fowl has been cooked, provided it includes fresh raisins from Syrian Damascus.

CHAPTER IV

Treatment of Urinary Incontinence not Due to Heat in the Kidneys

Dislocation of a vertebra is followed by perpetual micturition, a disorder not easily to be cured. However, rough massage to the loin and application of balsam, mustard with sulphur water, these do good: and if the bladder sphincter is relaxed so that the urine always passes, purge with mint and rhubarb. Foment the loins with rough red wine mixed with sage, rue, cypress, red roses, pine-nuts, oak and alum: and inunct the perineum, kidneys, hips and loins with oil of ben, flax, spikenard, mastic, and rue. Several agents bring relief: they include the brain of eagle, the kidneys, brain and testicles of nimble hare: the bladder of pig and goat, fierce bull and mild sheep, the lining of kid's and cockerel's gullet, tongue of goose, and mouse droppings, incense, myrrh and cyperus, myrobalan and calamint and mint and ewe's milk taken with pink sugar: alder and preserve of smooth coriander seed. Let a variety of substances be tested and their nature reported. Let the food be dry and sparse: roast pigeon or whatever birds have good juices, hazel and chestnut and the mast from Jove's spreading trees, and heavy matured red wine: for thin white wine is harmful, as is whey that moistens the kidneys and other things like radishes, cucumbers and melons, and drinking of much water and the frequent use of fruit.

CHAPTER V

Treatment of Inflammation of the Kidneys

When the kidneys become severely inflamed, prepare a cool enema to soothe the bowel: and then open a vein, the basilic first, not once but repeatedly. And if there is persistent heaviness and throbbing pain, fever and burning fire, it is very useful to swallow ordinary cassia and a cool apozeme that soothes the kidneys: for which take wood-sorrel and ordinary sorrel, dog's-tooth, asparagus and purslane, the seeds of melon, cucumber, lettuce, gourd, with the red berries of winter-cherry and dusky flowers of violet with water-lily: and in this drink dissolve syrups of sugar with juice of limes, violets and pomegranates. Rub the loins with ointment of oxyrhodium and poplar: foment with juices of nightshade, plantain, rose and lettuce mixed with penetrating vinegar, and the right amount of grains of camphor.

Use frequently fat broths of butter, asparagus, verjuice from early grapes, and flesh of calf with sorrel and succulent kid. But honey, pepper, and salt are harmful, as is that liquor said to be created by Semele's son. But give liquorice water with dog's-tooth, sorrel and juice of limes: if the pain presses fiercely and is not relieved by these, immerse in a warm bath. Water by itself is helpful, but it is more effective to add camomile, mallow, red roses and linseed: and if the arm has already been bled to excess, open the veins at the knee or ankle.

CHAPTER VI

Treatment of Abscess of the Kidney

Abscess of the kidney is disclosed when pus is seen in the urine: and cure, if it occur at all, is late. For this, first take black cassia daily: then open the elbow vein and next the saphenous: and an enema will cool and soothe the bowel. Frequently inunct the loin with poplar ointment and cerate of Galen, and foment as we have already told for diabetes. Terebinth is especially suited to cleanse and close the ulcer. But when the fever has taken hold, dark cassia with syrup of violets, pomegranate, myrtle and rose is helpful: and it is well to add water of lettuce, endive, roses, plantain and barley to make a julep. White wine is harmful unless the forces are depleted: let tisane and hydromel be drunk. Those herbs that stimulate the urine are harmful: therefore avoid wild celery, fennel and the like: but infuse together chicory, lettuce and chervil. The cream of barley is a useful food, and flesh and broth of chickens, and a meagre diet is best. However, if the disease be long, abandon this for easily digested flesh of turtle-dove and pigeon, fowl and fat capon and thrush: and it does not harm to drink the juice of fishes such as pike, perch, trout and carp nourished in the Seine, barbel and the sea-dragon or weever, red mullet, sole, the turbot that gives so much pleasure at state banquets, and our mighty sturgeon, allice-shad, and wrasse that is grateful to the palate: all cooked with sweet butter, of which that of Vanvre is most palatable.

CHAPTER VII

Treatment of Renal Pain or Calculus

When constant heaviness and pain are accompanied by the several signs already mentioned, stones are located in the kidney. Frequent use of an enema and suppository relieve the bowel: and if the veins are swollen, open the basilic first or else at the knee or ankle. And with this give by mouth syrup of jujube, mallow, violet, maidenhair and black cassia: and Calabrian manna or lenitive or senna and rhubarb to drink in water of winter-cherry or of pimpernel: and clear terebinth, if washed, can be given by itself or sometimes mixed with darkish marrow: and purge with cassia or diaprune or diaphenicum, mildly laxative, if the phlegm is harmful and the subject vigorous. Infusions that relieve are made with red chickpeas and hop, mallow and marshmallow, asparagus, veal and kid: and use fresh butter softened with sugar, and juice freshly expressed from sweet almonds, with white wine or tisane or pure water. The use of fomentations, poultices and liniments is excellent: for liniment, take oil of sweet almond, scorpion and camomile and rabbit-fat: make pultices of mallow or herbs mixed with the outer fat of pigs: and as fomentation, give mallow root and cyperus. Immerse the patient often in warm baths containing camomile and linseed in a sachet; and let the fluid drunk be such as to excite and dislodge the stone, that is, wild celery, fennel, parsley, burdock, birch, squill, rock samphire and stinging-nettle, radish, broom, iris, both kinds of star-thistle, yellow limes, juniper and laurel and many others, together with jew-stone and dissolved or powdered stone of lynx. The stone is fragmented by gums obtained from such trees as larch, fir, peach and cherry, or the water or oil distilled from stones of such trees as cherry or wild peach. And you may use ash of pigeons' feathers, blood of goat and buck burnt with their hide, and calcined horse's hoof, crab, cicada, earthworms and snail's shell: all to be taken as a syrup with lemon juice or white wine, or with sugar or a diuretic liquor. The fuming waters of sulphur and nitre are renowned: and whoever bathes in these or drains off many measures passes much urine: and if he has voided stone and gravel and feels relieved of his intolerable pain, he can return home happy and healthy: provided that, having been cleansed by a good physician, he observes a careful regime of food and drink.

CHAPTER VIII

Treatment of Bladder Stone

All to do with the cure of a kidney stone applies equally to a stone in the bladder: but the latter is longer-lasting and its remedies more devious, so that their effect is blunted. It is very difficult to disrupt a stone, unless it be extremely small. Purge often with powerful remedies: open the popliteal vein and the saphenous too if swollen. The various agents renowned for emptying out fluid or breaking up the stone are suitable for use: thus, powdered jewstone may be given with terebinth, or the stone contained in sponges and that from lynx's urine if it is hardened: and cassia with powdered camphor, or benedict with rhubarb and diaphenicum to swallow. Burnt glass, ashes of hare and wagtail, drunk in thin wine or oxymel: or the blood of young kid reduced to powder, oil of vitriol, the fluid distilled from metals, cinnamon water and infused lignum vitae: schoenanthum and wood of aloes and a due amount of nard, and galingale in water with seeds of juniper, laurel and ivy: warming bishopweed, wild carrot, mallow and cooling limes: cook all these with sugar and powdered bark of cinnamon to yield a delicate and aromatic fluid which, when drunk, avails to fragment the hard stone. And with a silver syringe, inject into the bladder water of iris, birch and saxifrage, artemisia, with radish and juice of lemon to wear away the stone. Rub into the groin and perineum a liniment made of oil of scorpion, fat of goose and rabbit. But if this has no effect, and the offending stone is not overcome, nothing is left but to cut the bladder with an instrument: and, that the disorder should not recur, avoid milk and sweet drinks made from milk, nor take any cheese, shun salted meats of goat and ox and goose and duck, or any bird that frequents lake, river or marsh: and scaleless fish from marsh and mud like slimy eels and tench, or even sumptuous lamprey: or yeastless uncooked bread mixed with sand and ash. Rice, too, is forbidden and beans and lentils except for chickpeas, and all vegetables, and must or dark wine and beer or muddied dirty water, or any food or drink that is foul or full of sticky juice. But well-baked leavened bread is good, prepared with dill and fennel: and also good are well-dressed partridge, capon, fowl and pheasant and rabbit fed on juniper: and turtle-dove and the famed wagtail and the thrush and other birds that fly in the fields. And make a habit of flesh of wether and young calf, and of scaled fishes and all we have mentioned in connection with the management of abscess of the kidney: and drink fine wine, sparkling and white, or oxymel or sugared water, and water infused with liquorice and dog's-tooth is recommended. Dates and raisins, fragrant pippins, stoned plums, strawberry and cherry, cooked pear, peach and fig: all these are good. But avoid harmful excess of food and drink: for ill fortune is his who indulges in rich food and gorges overmuch. Work before meals: all effort after eating is dangerous.

CHAPTER IX

Treatment of Inflammation of the Bladder

When the bladder is attacked by inflammation and swells rapidly, let an enema be given often to rid the bowel of faeces. Give cassis and diaprune and psillium as laxatives, Calabrian manna, rhubarb, cold seeds infused with sorrel, mallow, lettuce, asparagus and sweet-seeded fennel. Open a vein, first the basilic, then at the bend of the knee or at the ankle. Inject into the bladder plantain liquor, rosewater, warm houseleek water, lest the cold stifle the heat and gangrene destroy the part. Rub oxyrhodium into the pubes, moisten the patient and give a bath, and make a drink of lemons cooked with sugar and let the meat be veal and fowl and capon.

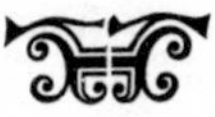

CHAPTER X

Treatment of Strangury and Dysuria

When the strangury, brought on the bladder by excessive cold, impairs the power to retain the urine, strengthen with thyme, origanum, calamint and rosemary, mint, marjoram: all made into a fomentation for penis and perineum. And make a liniment of oil of dill, rue, camomile, white lilies and of dead scorpion: or what is expressed from fragrant balsams. But first give a suppository or enema of salt, honey and olive oil cooked with the herbs listed above. Valuable are earthworms, woodlice and the ashed genitals of ferret, made into tablets with ten times as much sugar, to take by mouth. Or introduce into the urethral opening bed-bug, or an oiled wax candle, or a sound or catheter. It is good to take white wine often, whether the dysuria is due to weakness of the bladder or to wind: but for burning urine, pain, phlegmon, ulcer or abscess, after an enema open the basilic vein and then the saphenous. Black cassia is helpful, as is tragacanth: and frequent emulsions made from sweet almond and cold seeds, the seeds of henbane and white poppy with much sugar, to be drunk at midnight. The fluid of liquorice water boiled with raisins, with whey and cream of barley and milk of ass or grazing goat, relieves the pain, whether drunk or injected in the bladder: and prescribe syrup of jujube, violet, poppy, lemon: and immerse in a warm emollient bath: and give broths of tender veal and kid boiled with fowl and cool and tender herbs.

CHAPTER XI
Treatment of Ischuria

When the passages of bladder or kidney are narrowed or obstructed, see if there is a stone, blood-clot, phlegmon, thick humour, pus or some serous humour: and if there is a stone or phlegmon or pus, aim at a cure as has been related above. It is possible to dissolve a clot and open the passage by means of emollients. Thus, prepare an enema of birch, mallow, fat of tripes: sweet butter with sugar is a soothing drink with almond juice and wine: and use all that has a good effect on severe nephritis, such as terebinth mixed with marrow, cassia, diaprune, manna, senna, infused berries of the winter-cherry, the fruit of jujube with parsley seed and fennel, and mallow. And make a poultice of wall-pellitory, violet, linseed, marshmallow root and vesicants and fine yellow nightshade – the fruit infused with water, incense, chalk, the fat of pig and rabbit: and apply to the loins and hairy pubis. If this is ineffective, open the popliteal vein, moisten the body often or give hot baths: and search to see if anything is concealed within the bladder, pass a catheter to evacuate any stagnant urine: if there is a festering swelling, inject an emollient and evacuate the pus, cleanse a genital ulcer and strengthen the injured part with supportive liquors. And if there is proud flesh or callus, reduce this with a caustic, very cautiously, using powdered zinc oxide, lead and burnt alum. If the paths are obstructed by thick cold humour, inject warm water of origanum, fennel, wild celery and rock samphire to loosen them.

CHAPTER XII

Treatment of Priapism, or Satyriasis

The disease of satyriasis, also known as priapism, is to be cured by vomiting and bland enemas, and opening first the basilic vein and then the saphenous: and if the cause is a hot spirit that enters the penile orifice and makes it tense and turgid, then macerate purslane in cassia water with wild rhubarb and cold psillium confection, and introduce it very hot into the colon to relax the bowel. And warm water of lettuce and water-lily is to be drunk, with added syrup of violet and pomegranate. Rub in the groin and penis with rose-oil, violet and water-lily, or with Rhazes' ointment of white poplar. It is useful to add camphor, which restrains frenzied venery. Bind lead sheets around the loins and, if the cause of priapism is the wind, mix greens of rue and mustard in the diet: and make a mattress of the herb called agnus castus.

CHAPTER XIII

The Diet for Those Unable to Fulfil Their Marital Duties and for Those of Celibate Habit

If a husband performs badly, in that his sexual organ is lax and passive, let his diet be of good broths like turtle-dove and thrush, pheasant, pigeon, fowl and capon, blackbird and cockerel's testicles, and eggs of tender partridge: and add to these chickpeas, beans, pine-nuts, onions, asparagus, nuts of Cinara amula, root of wild parsnip and fennel, sweet almond, raisins if fresh, seed of colewort, dill and flax, the herb satyrion and leek, all kinds of shellfish, oysters especially, testes of fox and skunk, the organ of the stag, amber and musk, milk boiled with sugar, and the clove-pink. Let restoratives be often swallowed, and satyrion as antidote. Rub in castor oil around the penis: and the flanks with powdered pepper, myrrh and grains of musk as may be required. Let him keep a good table and drink perfumed wine. So much for husbands. As for the celibate, black bread and thin wine suffice, with water of lettuce soaked in vinegar, scaled fish, cherries, plums and pears, and all that unfits for love and war.

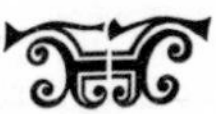

CHAPTER XIV

Treatment of True Gonorrhoea

If there is a flow of semen that is undesired and involuntary and nothing to do with sexual frenzy, it must be suppressed as soon as possible so that the body should not slowly waste. Sorrel and melon and gourd, spinach-beet, purslane, lettuce, the down of roses and especially the saffron flower: of these prepare a water and converse: and collect together poppy, staghorn fern, the three sandalwoods, coral, camphor, plantain and cool water-lily, to suppress the semen with their cold: and dry rue, hemp, calamint and mint resolve and dissipate what great heat has engendered. Take seeds of hemp and lettuce, rue, powder of coral and stag's horn, and make into tablets with ten times as much sugar, with a little rosewater or juice of mint, that weighs a dram, to be taken before meals. And smear the region of the loins with ointment of red sandalwood, Armenian bole, wax and oil of green myrtle: and bind round with leaves of rue or agnus castus or with lead sheets if the condition is severe, to draw the heat away from the kidneys. Make a drink with sugar of lettuce leaves, purslane, blackberry, cold seeds and flower of water-lily and juice of pomegranate. The diet should be meagre, so that cold in the testes suppresses the semen: and the water drunk should taste of quenched iron and heated stones. Let the air breathed be dry and cool, and the work be hard, and the clothes stained and dirty, so as to discourage and repel love's fastidiousness and render the sperm frequent and feeble.

CHAPTER XV

Treatment of Virulent Gonorrhoea

When the seminal discharge tautens the penis and the poison is accompanied by fierce pain, do not try to suppress it but first give a bland purge of manna and rhubarb to drink, or else the lenitive or terebinth or cassis can be taken often. Bleed from the knee or ankle vein. An emulsion is indicated containing the cold seeds known as pine-nuts, sweet almonds with white sugar and barley or plantain water: or perhaps syrup of water-lily, mallow and violets. To damp the burning of the penis, bathe it with warm milk or water. But if the case is not straightforward and the destructive poison results from impure intercourse, seek what is required to banish it: such as china root, wild celery, sarsaparilla, marrow, powdered lignum vitae, all of which dispel the poison by exciting sweating. And I advise comforting broths of the flesh of young kid and fowl, calf and young pigeons, with chervil, tart sorrel, bland lettuce, the plant called bugloss: and tisane of dog's-tooth or infused china root or sarsaparilla.

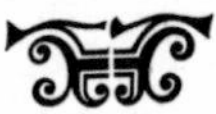

CHAPTER XVI

Treatment of Venereal Disease

The cure of the shameful venereal plague is by no means certain, seeing that its cause is obscure. However, this poison, through the humours, softens the marrow and the bones, a pollution born of seed: but if the measure of the poison is not properly assessed, it will return in much worse case: and this was well-known to famous authors, the earlier physicians like Machaon, who enquired into its nature, temperament and the abundant humour in which the poison lurks, so as to expel it with their art. It is well to infuse a drink of senna, hops, whey and bugloss with violets and fumitory: or hamech made up with lenitive may be given first. And if phlegm is burdensome, cleanse with white agaric, and then open a vein: and if the humour is dry, a warm bath softens the skin, opening the pores so that the poison is expelled in the sweat: and this is aided by scabious and cardoon, and the tormentil that dislodges the humours, fragrant balsam, juniper, the ash that will not suffer a reptile in its shade, box and many others that the earth produces in our clime. China root is best, and sarsaparilla is to be recommended, and infused lignum vitae to drink: but if the venom insinuates itself to attack the heart and brain, give alchermes, mithridatics, synthesis, Fernel's remedies and theriac as aids, together with conserve of roses, rosemary, bugloss, balm and borage, powdered precious stones and amber. Purge often with a variety of purges, so that the humours of this plague do not become attached but the residual malignant vapours are sweated out: and if this has no effect, though usually it restores to health, follow with mercurial inunction until foul saliva is expectorated. And while this is being applied to the body, let sarsaparilla, guaiac or china-root liquor be drunk to get rid of the poison the mercury induces: and if, as may be, this inunction is not tolerated, gain your effect with Vigo plaster on the arms and legs, for this promotes the salivary flow. And prepare pills of mercury with musk and scammony, rhubarb and gold, and triturate with flour moistened with lemon juice, and prescribe one to be swallowed daily: and it is considered that one of the remedies active against the disease is fennel water, of which drink an ounce a week, and half-an-ounce of aqua vitae. And the venereal contagion is lessened by perfumed pastilles of ladanum with cinnabar, mastic, incense, styrax, gum of juniper and aromatic flag: and those remedies are advised that secure evacuation of foul humours by the mouth and bowel and by sweating through the skin, such as infusions of lignum vitae and sarsaparilla. And now we touch briefly on the matter of diet. To bear up well until the end of the disease one must eat well, and that of flesh of kid and partridge, fowl and capon, turtle-dove, young hare and tender pigeon, more satisfactory if roasted: and of bread well-baked and spiced with dill or salt, and take tisane of china-root. But if the mercury induces excessive salivation, abandon meat for cooked prunes and jellied broths or eggs: and then, when the fury has spent itself, resume full nourishment, restore vigour with old wine, so that the body regains warmth and strength.

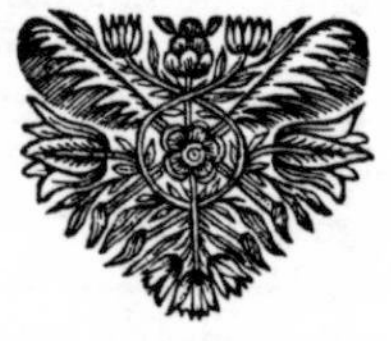

BOOK TEN

Preface

Now that I am left with this final work, support me, Holy Daughter and Mother of God: and You, of all women, can succour with your aid, that this work should supply remedies for women's ills, since You gave birth to an eternal Sun.

CHAPTER I

Hysterics, or Uterine Remedies

Cool remedies to suppress excessive menses are water-lily and cytisus and the astringent flower of the wild pomegranate, purslane evergreen, blackberry and plantain, sumach seed, ashes of burnt stag's horn and Indian ivory. But to provoke and warm the menses, take camomile, balm, betony and aristolochus, artemisia, horehound, the wood sorrel, the thyme bees browse on, noble polium of high mountains, basil, wild thyme, ornamental lilies, parthenia and dittany, origanum, trefoil and hazelwort, savin, pennyroyal, hartwort, calamint and rue, corncockle seed, black lovage root, peony, iris, water germander, madder and cyperus and the herb called gentian, bdellium, styrax, liquid amber, artichoke and myrrh, opopanax of course, the fragrant resins of sagapenum and galbanum, and beaver's testicles: all these favour the menstrual flow and encourage labour. And if the uterus is feeble, invigorate with the snakeweed's twisted cord, and the pale fluid of the poplar, and electrum known as yellow amber, and caryophyllum, nutmeg and mace, costmary, angelica, nard, the aromaric reed and benzoin, styrax, fragrant musk and amber.

CHAPTER II

Treatment of Unnatural Suppression of the Menses

If pain is caused by suppression of the menses, seek the cause. If it is due to worry, work, over-repose and slothful sleep, to sweat or diarrhoea or loss of blood, let these be halted. If it is fat or clot, dissolve it: if a fleshy growth, cut it away. If it is a slow humour, apply hot fomentations to dislodge it and purge with hyeris, diaphenicum and subtilizing herbs such as fennel, hyssop, calamint and pennyroyal. Pastilles of myrrh often succeed in opening the menses, as does chickpea broth with parsley, buttery, veal and capon, with saffron added. It is well to drink water tinctured with madder or with mint, also weak Sabine wine and water of cinnamon bark is excellent: and sugar, bark of cinnamon and wine squeezed through an hippocras bag. And perfume may excite the menses: the aromas of marjoram and powdered laurel berries, juniper, nard with styrax, benzoin. And hip-baths may be effective, with flowers of camomile and rosemary, marjoram, catmint, origanum, thyme. Rub in the groin and pubes with oil of nutmeg, ladanum and juice of balsam mixed with wax: or make a pessary of mercurial powder, fragrant musk or amber. And if the cause of the disorder is thick obstruction of the uterine veins, open the basilic and then the veins at the knee or ankle: but before this, inject a gentle clyster in the anus to purge out the excess humour, and then purge bile or phlegm. Follow with baths, in which infuse mallow and marshmallow, camomile, fennel and fragrant balsam.

CHAPTER III

Treatment of Pallor in Young Girls

If pallor in girls is due to cooling of the skin by drink, or to excess of uncooked food, it is well to drink wine mixed with water or wine of absinth, and roast birds are good to eat. It is meet to take pills of hyeris and ruffi to purge the bile and phlegm that attack the stomach, and expel them in the bowel. And make pastilles of mint and nard, galingale and cassia and yellow rhubarb and add them to the white agaric and pale roses to make a sugar syrup. Take tablets containing powdered iron with delicate herb margaret, mastic powder, compounded alchermes, gemstone and agreeable galenic. Foment the stomach with warm cyperus, wormwood and odorous reed. If there has been excessive use of pepper, cloves, nutmeg or salt, the girl should swallow broths or butter with flesh of kid or calf and leaves of purslane and fresh mallow. There is no better purge than black cassia and tepid bathing should be frequent. Let tisanes or cool fluids with bread be drunk: and if the pallor is because the menses fail, we have already told how to bring these on.

CHAPTER IV

Treatment of the Hysteric Suffocation, or Furor Uterinus

In suffocation of the uterus, first test for any sign of life by inserting powdered pyrethrum or hellebore using a feather in the nostril, pull out the hair from the lower parts: if the hysteric neither breathes nor moves nor feels, but lies as if lifeless, still, if life persists, bind the limbs with ligatures and especially massage the legs. Expose to foetid odours, rue, galbanum, castoreum, spurge, gagates, and burnt hair, horn or feather. And it is helpful to exhibit, to the part shameful to speak of, such fragrances as musk and bombax, civet, gallia renowned for sweetness, alypum and amber, wood of aloes, cloves, mace and styrax, also ladanum. The oils of lily, costmary, spikenard and laurel, mixed with amber, are very helpful. But if the humour is too thick, purge with suppositories or enemas: and then give hyeris and diaphenicum to drink, or rosemary preserve with the agaric fungus, made into a bolus with terebinth. If the blood is at fault, open the vein at the knee. If excess of bad seed is produced by the womb, whether in a nun, widow or virgin or the sick, rub in the pudendal parts with oil of water-lily: let her smell camphor and green rue with hemp. Purslane with lettuce is helpful in the diet, but otherwise meals should be small and delicate: and let her lie on agnus castus. The frenubile virgin, joined in marriage, engages frequently in coupling. If it is the uterine fury, that is also curable by art: but since the heat is greater in this case, bleed more freely, give cool drinks and food and syrups, suppository and enemas: and let syrup of violet with cassia and water-lily be drunk.

CHAPTER V

Treatment of Excessive Menstrual Flow

For troublesome excess of menstrual flow, open the basilic vein widely, and cup beneath both breasts using much flame: and tightly bind and warm the hands and often massage: and, for fluids, prescribe a draught of cool plantain water with pomegranate and syrup of myrtle. And give pastilles of powdered amber and spodium and Lemnian earth with Armenian bole: or powdered coral, jasper, dragon's blood and haematite. And you may add conserve of roses, water-lily and cassidony, compound with myrtle liquor and sugar, taking a portion of chestnut size before meals daily. A longish pessary of wool and silk-cotton, soaked in fluid of willow and plantain, is used to fit the genitals: and the parts around are rubbed with oxyrhodium. Philonium is an antidote, and rest, and inspissate and suppress the flow when other measures fail. The woman with excessive menses should lie quietly and let her diet be meagre: the juice of a roast is laudable, with red currant and pomegranate juice or the fruit of thorny barberry. If the veins stand out, bleed freely: if the bone is dark and black, so is the humour: and if it is green or yellow, there is bile; and whiteness is a sign of phlegm. Thus there is a remedy for each occasion: if languor persists, retain the flow, but continue to evacuate the humour if the patient is vigorous.

CHAPTER VI

Treatment of the White Flux

When there is a uterine discharge not of the ordinary colour, the woman has a flux that it is proper to arrest with those astringents listed elsewhere. If the flow be red, open the elbow vein: if pale, expel it with yellow rhubarb or some such purge: a black humour is to be purged with hops and senna and the so-called hamech: the antidote to phlegm is diaphanicum and delicate with agaric orally. If the blood is serous, hasten its outflow from the kidneys with fennel and white celery, so that thicker blood may be secreted and settle in the uterus. Drink sudorifics such as sarsaparilla and guaiac, devil's-bit and warming cardoon to open the skin's pores and let out filth. If the cause of the disorder be thickness of the skin, it is wise to rub with a linen cloth gently and again. Counter the flow and discharge the residue with water of equisetum and hypocistis, the infused flower and fruit of blackberry, pomegranate fruit and amaranthus flowers. And prepare a tablet to be taken before meals of white ivory and red coral powdered, rosewater and sugar. If the passage of an acrid humour is painful, ass's milk with pink sugar comforts and a tisane with rice cooked in milk. If an ulcer soils the genitals, clean carefully with warm water and rub in with oil of roses, myrrh and quince: and, that the flow should not return, give a bitter, hot and windy diet, encourage work and baths, give what is purgative and diuretic. The diet should be as we have already said.

CHAPTER VII

Treatment of Weakness of the Uterus

The uterus is weak is there is excess of phlegm due to raw vegetables or fruit or to the water. Take fowl, partridge, turtle-dove, quail, pheasant and young woodcock: and let bark of cinnamon mixed with sugar-water be drunk, and old wine or hydromel. Prescribe herb margaret before meals, and tablets of fragrant roses and gemstones afterwards. Take rose and grains of civet, amber, musk, styrax, spikenard, galingale and odorous rush and amber from the poplar tree: mix all these together, triturate into powder and burn in the fire, shape into a pessary and insert into the entry of the private parts. If the cause of this weakness is frequent labour or miscarriage, or cold or phlegm, the treatment is the same: but restrain the woman from all movement and seclude her from all grief. Dancing is harmful, and to be borne by fast horses in a carriage, whether heat or cold is the cause. But preserve of water-lily with coral suppresses heat.

CHAPTER VIII

Treatment of Phlegmon and Erysipelas of the Uterus

If there is pain in the loins and pubis, and a hot and heavy swelling in the uterus, evacuate the bowel with enemas composed of cool emollient herbs: or mix honey, oil of violet and fresh butter. Open a flow from veins at the knee or ankle, and repeat as vigour is regained: bind the limbs and massage to divert blood from the uterus. Use syrup of violet and water-lily mixed with water as a drink. Take cassia often and Calabrian manna, rhubarb with whey and senna, black tamarind, lettuce and purslane, to purge the hidden bile and expel all heat from within the womb. And if it does not altogether cease, foment the loins, groins, pubes and cervix with water of sedum, lettuce, roses, and use liniment of oil of water-lily, quince and roses. And if the heat does not yield even to these, immerse the woman's body in warm water. Let the food be moist and the simples cold: water is best to drink, but adding cinnamon and sugar does no harm: but if the woman is accustomed to the use of wine, and water is not well digested, let her drink wine diluted with water: but if the sacred fire devours down below, give pure water only and apply cool water to the private parts. Calm her complaints with gentle speech, and give syrup of water-lily and poppy to induce drowsiness.

CHAPTER IX

Treatment of Abscess of the Uterus

If the discharge of hot stinking pus from the uterus indicates the presence of an abscess or ulcer, give cleansing injections down below of warm and honeyed whey, to which add juice of psillium and plantain, lettuce and purslane, rose-juice with metrenchyta liquor, into the foul cavity of the uterus. And dry up and strengthen with whatever opens and dislodges poison by adding alum, ointment of lead and diapompholyx and white lead: the first red, the second white. Cassia with rhubarb and foreign senna are to be drunk, and frequently insert a suppository or enema into the bowel. Dry food favours discharge of pus and humour from the uterus and adjacent parts: for liquor, take barley-water and pink sugar, hydromel and cinnamon with bark and sugar.

CHAPTER X

Treatment of Scirrhus of the Uterus

If a scirrhus is located in the uterus, give a liquid diet to stop its generation by foul humour: or roasts if time allows and the country is very damp: or if the bowel is relaxed, all juices are excellent, the flesh of fowl, calf and capon, kid, plump thrush and fleet hare: prescribe liquorice and raisins infused in water and take more water with the wine. Aid discharge of the thick dark humour from the bowel with frequent broths, or plums and raisins, hop, lettuce, sorrel and senna. Soften the site of scirrhus with wool moistened with lanolin, oil of almond, dill or lily, the fat of fowl, duck, pig, goose or fox or marrow of deer: and prescribe mallow with figs and marshmallow, bear's-breech as fluid, and fragrant styrax, resin and terebinth, the exudate of larch and fir, thyme and famed Libyan ammoniac: bdellion, opoponax, virgin wax and the malodorous juice of galbanum.

CHAPTER XI

Treatment of Cancer of the Uterus

The cure of cancer is not given to Machaon's secret art, and cancer of the uterus fathoms the depths of ill: yet it may be alleviated by various remedies, so that it does not grow or spread. First purge the black humour in the bowel with senna and whey mixed with cassia and manna, filicula and plum. If the woman's veins are full of thickened blood, bleed first from the basilic vein, then at the knee or ankle. If the black blood appears as swollen haemorrhoids, attack these by opening with an instrument or with yellow leeches: and that the liver should not generate a foul black humour and relay it by the veins to spleen and body, the best diet is broth, but not too much, of capon, turkey, the tender flesh of calf and kid cooked in butter or solidified as jelly, or the expressed juices of their flesh: and snails and crayfish especially. For thirst, give water only, mixed with a little wine if you think fit. For health, proffer tisane of barley containing liquorice, clustered grapes and juicy raisins: and prescribe fragrant apple juice and its royal-savoured syrup, and often conserve of bugloss and of hyacinth, and tablets of precious herb margaret. Obtain the oil of frog and crayfish: or ointment of pompholyx and lead: rose-juice, nightshade and henbane and juices of plants like houseleek: and add warm milk if there is a foul malignant ulcer, and prescribe whey often or tisane of cream of barley.

CHAPTER XII
Treatment of Fleshy Mole

The shapeless so-called fleshy mole, if allowed to remain hidden in the womb, usually persists for several years, sometimes so long as not to be surrendered before the time of death. And this disease is caused by retention of the menses, or because the man's semen is diseased or weak. The woman should shun coitus, so as not to aggravate the humour: so that the menses should flow and the mole be at the same time resolved or cast down, open the basilic vein or the cubital, then the popliteal or the saphenous at the ankle: then purge with white agaric fungus, senna, catmint, maidenhair, hyssop and betony, thyme and fennel and both kinds of hyeris. And give baths containing camomile and mallow with laurel leaves and linseed: and foment the groins and pubes with sage infused with polium and wine: make pessaries with oil of dill, iris or lily, butter and deer's marrow or juice of marjoram and old wine. Apply to the lower belly a poultice made of roots of marshmallow and white lilies recooked with hydromel and fat of goose and pig: Jove's dittany from Crete and castoreum drunk with fragrant wine, or water of parthenium or other herbs that induce menstrual flow may dislodge the mole and restart the menses. But if this does not happen, and if pastilles of myrrh are also unsuccessful, take the mirror for the womb and insert it to see where the mole is, at the os or sides or confined above, and note its site, that the surgeon may see it and remove it with his art.

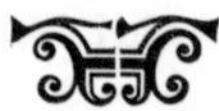

CHAPTER XIII

Treatment of True or Simple Gonorrhoea in Women

When discharge soils the genitalia without itching, often involuntarily and without the woman feeling it, prescribe rhubarb and cassia together, or with lettuce, sorrel, hemp and rue, lenitive and chicory or senna: and if the body abounds in perverse humours, give often pink pomegranate syrup, water-lily, myrtle: and quince before meals is costive in these cases. Take oil of water-lily, oxyrhodium and Armenian bole and make a liniment for the loins, midbelly and hairy pubes: and of powdered Cyreniac carab beetle, mastic and rose apply the vapour to the genitals. Let the diet be delicate and meagre, and pink sugar-water should be drunk: and consult those places where I have dealt with the treatment of gonorrhoea and satyriasis, the one oppressive to women, the other to men.

CHAPTER XIV

Treatment of Virulent Gonorrhoea in Women

A persistent foetid thick discharge emerges from the cervix of the uterus, white or green or yellow, stinging and often ulcerating the skin, a foul poison believed to be an outcome of the pox. And, that it should not spread and infect the uterine parts, give whey and senna or syrup of violets and cassia: and cold seeds, the cream of barley and sweet almonds as julep with white sugar, to be often drunk with honey. Bleed at the ankle lest a swollen vein carry infection upward in the blood. Bathe the ulcer with warm cow's milk mixed with plantain water and inject metrenchymata into the vaginal cavity until it overflows to soothe any hidden ulcer. But if it is not so soothed, prescribe a drink of china root and sarsaparilla: and if success is still delayed, inunct the woman with mercurial ointment until the throat becomes moist and swollen and the tongue protrudes and much phlegm is discharged from the mouth, fouling all with its unpleasant odour.

CHAPTER XV

Treatment of Inflation or Tension of the Uterus

If the womb is swollen, tense and sonorous with wind, to arrest this give a diluent enema with infused seeds of fennel, wild carrot with hyeris and oil of pristine laurel, nard, dill, rue or iris. Prepare fomentations with horehound, pennyroyal, fragrant thyme and polium: and rub the groins, pubis, flanks and back with oil of nard, laurel and pepper and powder of gum terebinth with a little wax. If the cause of the flatus is crude humour lurking in the liver, and it is feared that the harmful phlegm will not be expelled from the burdened part, prescribe remedies to discharge the phlegm: agaric fungus, diaphenicum, diacatharmus, benedict: and at the same time use the liniment described and foment the part. Irritate the skin to redness with fig, raisins and mustard, and apply many large cupping-glasses to the belly. Bathe in water infused with emollient herbs: mallow, flowers of camomile, those that subtilize and induce the menstrual flow like parsley, marjoram, calamint and parthenic. Insert into the vagina a finger lubricated with olive oil or butter or fat of goose or pig to break up any clot: and if the hand fails in this attempt, use a syringe to inject into the uterine cavity those emollient herbs called metrenchymata, to liquefy and release whatever clot the uterus contains: and if the disorder is caused by excess of blood, bleed moderately from the popliteal vein. Pigeons are fit birds to eat, and the food should be well-peppered, and the wine old and delicate, fragrant and sparkling: but if a crude humour engenders flatus that obstructs the flow of blood, the diet should be delicate and devoid of heat and the wine diluted with water.

CHAPTER XVI

Treatment of Hydrops of the Uterus

To arrest the swelling of the uterus by retained fluid, restore the red liver and the darker spleen to their former healthy state and re-establish the menstrual flow. If it is evident that bile dominates the body, draw it out with rhubarb and manna, and give colocynth and white agaric for the humour and fern and senna if it is black:

and for the fluid, give pale roses, diacatharmus and pastilles of colocynth known as alhandal. Then give enemas and suppositories often. Prescribe hyeris, elder, iris of course, and elder and a mixture of dill with two drachms weight of black hellebore, with honey and the oil of iris: these, known as metrenchymata, inject into the uterus, a juice that attracts water and mucus. And these are also dislodged by ointment of spurge applied to the belly, as well as poultices of snails and sulphur: and waters of sulphur, vitriol or nitre are helpful both in the bath-water and the drink.

CHAPTER XVII

Treatment of Ascent, Descent and Procidentia or Prolapse of the Uterus

To ensure that the uterus be not upwardly displaced, the woman should sniff the odours of galbanum, gagate, rue, burnt hair and all that is foul and foetid: and moisten the genitals with juice of marjoram and myrrh, ladanum, Nabathean incense, bland musk or civet, whatever has an overwhelming fragrance: and trickle Cyreniac gum into the os, so as to direct the Panchaian odours to the secret places below. But, that the uterus should not descend too far, keep it in place with a supportive pessary soaked in thin wine or red rosewater in which plantain has been infused: and foment the pubes with a sponge soaked in oxycrat. If it should chance to prolapse externally in a mighty fall, injuring the part, gently lift and replace it so that all is once again in its proper place. But that it should not recur, the woman should lie down with legs extended and one thigh crossed over the other, and prepare a pessary: but first foment with wool soaked in wine and juice of pomegranate and hypocistis: apply fragrant odours to the nose and stinking vapours to the shameful parts and large cupping-glasses to hips and belly, rubbing beforehand with royal oil of myrtle to tighten the parts. And, that the part should not be consumed by gangrene, give an enema at once and let her pass urine: and, having restored the uterus to its proper place, open an elbow vein, for fear that an attack of colic and diarrhoea might risk further prolapse. Her voice should not be heard, not should she cough or sneeze too often, and she should walk calmly and no more than necessary and repose with tranquil mind. Let the diet be sparse and delicate, also the wine. And she must submit to wear a cork pessary of oval shape, with thread appended, placed in the empty vagina, so that it can be withdrawn if the wishes to micturate or when she lies abed, and that the womb be retained at the right level and not suffer loss of its position: and coat the pessary with wax all over.

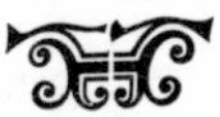

CHAPTER XVIII

The Management of Pregnancy

The woman who has just conceived should not be moved by anger, nor be depressed by grief or care or apprehension, nor carry heavy burdens or ride on horseback or in a carriage, nor dance or act in any violent manner, lest the infant drop hazardously from the womb. But her duties should be light, let her weave a wicker basket or spin wool or knit, work with a needle embroidering the shapes of men and animals: and if she seeks the country, she should walk at the pace of an old woman, or go on a soft litter, or be borne slowly on an ass. And if, after two months, she suffers discomfort in the stomach, thirst and anxiety, has nausea and vomiting, expectorates, is squeamish and averse to food, but goes chewing earth or shells of coals, things unsuitable for food, or salted victuals or vinegar, purge out the noxious humour with gentle purges such as manna, yellow rhubarb, senna, boiled in soft bland greasy broths, or lenitive, or those remedies that together draw out the humours. If the blood is too abundant, open the median or the basilic vein: but do not remove so much as to deprive the child of nourishment. The diet of a pregnant woman must be easy to digest and her wine well watered, for thus there is less risk of miscarriage: and that the uterus should not lose its power, place on the belly eagle-stone and Samian ware or yellow jasper, or the stone found in the hind's womb or belly, to ensure that the foetus does not move about: but remove this as the time of labour nears so that the womb may open speedily. It is useful to take tablets of abbatis before meals, or of the three sandalwoods, gemstones, rosewater and quince.

CHAPTER XIX

Remedies to Expel the Dead Foetus

When the dead infant cannot be expelled from the uterus, and if the menses have not recommenced and the woman's vessels are distended with much blood, remove the faeces with a suppository or strong enema, open a vein at the elbow or the ankle, purge with effective laxatives like agaric, diaphenicum, diacatharmus, and benedict. Prescribe water of dittany, fern and bramble, thyme, savin, horehound, germander, cantaury, pennyroyal, calamint and balm: or give galbanum and myrrh mixed with wine and pennyroyal and two drachms of castoreum: so that the dead but unborn child within the womb should not give rise to vapours that endanger its parent. Bind on the thigh the eagle-stone, jasper or Samian ware. The cyclamen, again, has such a corrupt and stinking odour as to induce abortion: and fumigate the private parts with myrrh, bothrys and fragrant calamus, sulphur, anchusa root and white alum. And if all this fails, and even wormwood cannot expel the foetus from the uterus, let the surgeon with his magisterial art extract it in pieces with hand and instruments.

CHAPTER XX
Remedies for a Difficult Labour

When a pregnant woman carries a live child in her womb and is apprehensive of difficulty in labour, if her time be near and if the bowels do not open freely but retain hard faeces within, expel them with suppository or enema and encourage the passage of urine from the kidneys. Let her consume broths infused with butter and mallow, coddled fresh eggs, pressed flesh of veal, partridge, capon and their jelly, above all the flesh of snails: and roast turtle-dove with juniper berries, green laurel, powder or bark of cinnamon: and let the wine be mixed with water. It is helpful to apply warm oil of camomile or almonds or white lilies to the uterus: the perfume of origanum, incense and benzoin will gradually induce the os to open. And when the pains are oft repeated and the open uterus pours forth its waters, the woman should stand up and be ordered to restrain her wind and powerfully exert herself to push the foetus downwards. Let her sniff pyrethrum to make her sneeze, and take relaxing hippocras whose taste restores declining vigour: or give cinnamon water, or water of saffron or white lilies. And if all these do not sufficiently dilate the os, and both child and mother are too weak for it to be expelled, prescribe wine and water mixed with dittany, or myrrh in pastilles: and undertake the same exertions as described above for extracting a dead child. As we have already said, there are many causes of a difficult labour: and these must be considered carefully in treatment lest death overtake both mother and child.

CHAPTER XXI

Remedies to Expel the Afterbirth or Chorion from the Uterus

If the membrane known as the chorion or afterbirth is retained within the uterus, whose orifice stays shut, insert a hand within lubricated with soft goose-fat or lard, butter or oil of camomile, lily or iris, to relax the os and extract the afterbirth by its matted fringes: but do this very cautiously so as not to pull out uterus with placenta, an ill beyond repair. And if it is not possible to manually extract this appendage from the uterus, perfume with aromatic odours from jars containing nard, cassia, iris, aromatic reed, gladdening Cyperus root, wormwood, dittany, polium, savin, ladanum, styrax, bdellium and benzoin. Give powdered hellebore often as sternutant to stimulate the uterus, and provoke it also with frequent suppositories of hyeris: and purge with those other powerful agents like white agaric or benedict in those waters used to induce the menstrual flow. If it seems that the woman has the same forceful pains she had in previous labours, give castoreum mixed with water of polium, thyme or pennyroyal, pastilles of myrrh, the leaves and expressed juice of parsley, or cassis, or famed infusion of wood of cinnamon: and use ointment of cyclamen and myrrh to rub the belly, and a pessary of the same with lathyrum, which usually expels the afterbirth from the uterus.

CHAPTER XXII

Treatment of Sterility Due to Various Causes

That woman does not conceive whose private parts are numb and cold and thick, dried up by excess heat or affected by too much moisture, or strictured without an opening. If it is cold that makes the uterus sterile, release the cold humour by giving remedies that dislodge the phlegm: give warming herbs like betony, polium, thyme, horehound, hyssop that induce the menses: or make pessaries of marjoram juice and the right amount of grains of musk: and preserve of sage, swallowed, makes fecund and prevents destruction of the foetus. Roast flesh is best, and best is watered wine. If the womb is burning hot and the heat must be dispelled, cassia is indicated and much relieves the fire, with purslane, lettuce, sorrel: and drink water often and infuse the meat with soothing herbs and bathe in sweet water and let life be tranquil and care-free. If excessive humour moistens, dry out with frequent exercise and prescribe a meagre diet of roast birds with bread twice-baked, salted or spiced with aniseed. Perfume the uterus with Sabaean incense, ladanum, myrrh, origanum, polium and thyme: but first dislodge the faeces from the bowel with suppository or enema, and bleed abundantly should it be necessary. If there is constriction, dilate and rub with goose-fat principally, fat of calf and stag's marrow. And there are other causes of sterility in women, to be treated carefully by contraries: but she may not be sterile, but married to a man who is impotent, or cannot sow fertile seed, so that then both must be investigated to see if both are healthy, or if there is any discrepancy in age or temperament or love or in production of the seed, and that they are neither idle nor labour to excess but keep a middle way. Their food should be easily cooked, their wine bland, let them enjoy raisins, the artichokes and asparagus that adorn our gardens, onions and turnips, leeks, fresh parsnips, horehound root, and obtain those best of shellfish, oysters. Let them live together quietly and not stuff their stomachs with too much food, lest they grow fat from excess of crude blood and therefore produce less seed. If they follow this regime, the woman will soon become fertile and bear a child.

CHAPTER XXIII

Treatment of Exanthemata

Children have a common disease which spreads as variable red spots, and the skin itself is often reddened unless conquered by our art.

Therefore, if the papules advance slowly and there is no fever, and the child has significant bad humour, remove the faeces from the bowel with enema or suppository. Give cardiac waters like devil's-bit, wood sorrel, scabious, lemons and bitter quince, which extrude the poison from the heart into the skin. The child should be kept in warm air, wrapped in many coverings, sheltered from all draughts, so that sweat and spots are expelled together: and let his aliment be frequent jellies, the juices pressed from meat, lettuce cooked in milk or butter, sorrel and bugloss. And give for drink pale lemon juice with sugar, prepare tisanes of lentils, figs and liquorice, seeds of fennel and lemon, which excite much sweat: and these can be cooked with figs and raisins. And if, before the spots appear, there is much diurnal fever, an unequal burden, it is because the poison is not exuded from the skin: remove the matter by opening a vein, but first give an enema. Prescribe Calabrian manna to drink, dissolved in broth of fowl or veal: and if the white skin is stained with various colours, do nothing unless there is choking and rasping breathlessness heralding a fatal outcome, an indication for opening the vein. Assess the strength as best you can: and it is as well to give a poor prognosis, full of anxiety: and do not bleed a child that is still at nurse lest, if the disease have a fatal outcome, you will be held responsible and your reputation and your art be sullied, profaned by insolence and frenzy.

CHAPTER XXIV

Treatment of Porphyra, or the Purple Fever

This fever, purple by name and nature, colours our body red and is marked by purple mottling, terrifying in its new and strange malignity, such as to defeat our ancestor physicians until Apollo showed us how to attack it by providing us with a weapon. There were those with feeble pulse, tremor and torpor, confused and wavering, their urine thick and red, at times as thin as water: the faeces, ashen, yellow, white or green came stinking from the bowel. Treatment was with cardiacs, such as imperial drink, germander, devil's-bit, scabious, sorrel, cardoon, citraginis and wood sorrel and sugared acid juices of lemon, lime and pomegranate: and also theriac water and antidotes like mithridatum, alcherm, herb margaret, hyacinth. But these proved poor protection, the panting did not cease and fever persisted, nor was the air the sole cause of the illness: nor was the poison solely in the heart but also in the brain and a pestiferous humour in every part, not to be dispelled by hand or instrument. It was long debated whether its purple colour indicated that the blood was peccant, so that the swollen vein be opened: it was feared that, if the poison was released from within the body, it might wreak havoc, cause fainting and a feeble, small and irregular pulse: and this troubled the physician's mind. But it seemed more sensible not to underestimate the vital forces: rather, that the oppressed heart would revive after bleeding, and that the poison, leaving the internal parts, would no longer inflict its corruption on the body. So profuse bleeding was done from time to time, and purging, and the heart restored with cardiacs as we have said before, and sweating induced. Food was prepared to restore the forces: turtle-dove and thrush, cock and tender capon and young pigeons, cooked with digestives such as sorrel, bugloss and the like: and expressed meat juices and jellies, or liquor doubly distilled in vessels: with powder of bezoar and pearl and precious stones, ivory, horn of rhinoceros and unicorn and stag and fragrant amber, mixed together: and preserve of borage, water-lily, bugloss, violet and roses, all to be applied as a poultice to the heart: and cupping to be done at various sites, the skin scarified under a ruddy flame, and leeches applied to the vessels. And many persons recovered from this fearful ill, which formerly had immersed innumerable victims in the waters of the Styx.

CHAPTER XXV

Treatment of Gout

When a subtle and warm humour, flowing into the joints, causes acute vexatious pain, bleed on the side opposite to the pain: purge with a lenitive, manna or senna, and assuage the ardour by prescribing cool lettuce, plantain, chicory and rose waters, with syrup of pomegranate and myrtle. And to drink ass's milk and cassia is especially assuaging: and it gives new comfort to the part to apply a poultice at the site of pain, made of soaked bread infused with saffron, penetrating vinegar, the mucilaginous seeds of psillium, and oil of nightshade with earthworms and rose-oil. If the flow does not cease with these, and the pain persists sharp and severe, preventing sleep, infuse together milk and henbane leaves, or milk with opium, which produce numbing of the senses: and at night give barley-water: and the white fluid expressed from sweet almonds taken with sugar and white poppy seeds relieves and removes the pain and restores peaceful sleep. And then give the golden pill, and pills of wild rhubarb dissolved in water of lettuce or water-lily or syrup of violets, both together expelling the bile that causes pain within the joints. And if this does not relieve the flow of humour, infuse camomile, bugle, oak-galls, roses, mixed with dark wine: and apply a poultice of fresh cow-dung to the part: or use the materials for fomentation with butter and roses to rub into the groin. If the gout is due to phlegm, it is often purged into the bowel by pills of white agaric and other remedies that dislodge the phlegm: coction of the phlegm is best when it is attached to the parts and causing severe pain: so foment with origanum, melilot with camomile and roses, oil of fox or turpentine, and even smear with worms moistened with alder and ivy. Sage, elder, marjoram, germander, castoreum and ebulus and laurel berries are to be taken. The mucilage of seeds of fenugreek and oxycrat and honey remove the pain within three days, as does rubbing with the mucus of a snail. As for the nodules resulting from the phlegm, Podalirius possessed the remedy: however, some may still be cured by old cheese dissolved in broth of ham, by diachylon of Iris, mercurial Vigo plaster, or oil of ben with grease of pig and goose. For the sciatica, give ranunculus and cress, pine resin, terebinth, pitch and sulphur and pigeon's dung, all to be applied as blisters to the painful part. But first, induce vomiting and remove the faeces with an enema or with hyeris. Bleed in the arm, then at the knee: abandon Bacchus, offspring of Semele, and Cytherean Venus. Live a frugal life, and to drink water in place of wine will divert elsewhere the raging pains of podagra and dire chyragra.

CHAPTER XXVI
Treatment of Elephantiasis

It is barely possible to eliminate elephantiasis, once established in the parts or giving rise to cancer in the organs: however, the attempt was made by Podalirius, of whom the Muses sing. Give Calabrian manna frequently to drink, and Indian cassia and senna soaked in whey: or plums and raisins, in both of veal or kid. Open the veins, apply leeches to the blemishes to suck the black blood from various parts: attach cupping-glasses to extract a flow after scarifying the skin, and blisters to the swollen limbs. Give frequent warm baths to open the skin pores and release the vapour that makes the body drowsy and inert, to be replaced by a gentler vapour to warm the inner parts. And then hyeris with colocynth is useful, and hamech and pills of fumitory containing black hellebore: or, if you like, indigo or famed lapis lazuli. The food should be young turkeys, and our own cooks, capons and tender veal, which please when roasted in the acid juice of pomegranate, oxyacantha or red currant: or if they are boiled, it is more fitted to the disease to cook with sorrel, lettuce, plantain, violet, chicory, borage and bugloss. Eggs are good if fresh, and milk of almonds, and pink sugar mixed with cream of barley, and milk from the full teats of asses: and to eat an easily digested fish occasionally will do no harm: and barley bread. Salt and spices harm, as does the flesh of pig, deer, ass, rabbit and ox, cheese unless freshly made, beans and all vegetables, nor pears either unless cooked. If constipated, give apples, cherries, melon, lettuce and purslane with vinegar and delicate fruit of capers: the liquor of cooked apples aids, diluted with sugar-water, mixed with syrup of lemon, cassia and bark. Wine is unsuitable, and beer, and other thick juices, but instead infuse liquorice and raisins and mix syrup of violets with the resultant fluid. Our predecessors argued that castration was a way to health: but if this is not to the patient's liking, revive him with frequent baths and secure profuse sweating with sarsaparilla and inunct with mercurial ointment. But, because the poison is so deadly, use those remedies that are most indicated, such as the mithridatic antidote and theriac, filings of ivory and staghorn and green emerald: and let the patient drink wine in which a viper has died, or eat its flesh after cutting off the head, spiced with salt and leek and oil of dill, as Pergameus testified and Galen recommended. However, if this cure seems hazardous, and you shrink from the poison in the viper's flesh, give the broth in which a viper has been cooked to fowls and when their feathers fall give them to the patient: and this will enable a leper to abandon his old age and resume the tender flesh of youth.

In what French reign the author completed this book:

I finished this work when Louis XIII was King reigning over the French, and his august mother Regent, to the plaudits of the Senate, princes and the common people: whom I pray to be inclined to peace, and to protect the laws and religion which former monarchs have always cherished.

If these verses have displeased you, at least they have been my consolation: if pleasing, then I am content.

INDEX

Please note that all page numbers in *italics* denote "signs and causes", while those in **boldface** designate "treatment".